Myth Psychoanalysis

Myth Psychoanalysis: Freud, Lacan and Lévi-Strauss examines the human psyche through the theoretical lenses of three groundbreaking thinkers, exploring how humans craft their symbolic reality.

This innovative work treats the exemplary cases of Freud as myths, parallel to native myths in their structure and the knowledge they harbor. The book reviews what Freud, Lacan and Lévi-Strauss would say on various aspects of the human psyche, identifying commonalities and discrepancies while distilling truths that resonate through the intersection of their perspectives. Through twelve comprehensive chapters, the work explores creation myths, kinship relations, totemism, and the structural foundations of meaning-making in both clinical and cultural contexts. The author employs a storytelling style that brings to life fascinating narratives from native myths and psychoanalytic case studies, making complex theoretical concepts accessible through engaging examples and biographical insights.

This book is fascinating reading for psychoanalysts, mental health professionals, and those familiar with Freud, Lacan, or Lévi-Strauss who seek to enrich their knowledge and clinical application.

Yehuda Israely, Ph.D. is a psychologist, psychoanalyst and writer, winner of the Israeli Gefen award for original Sci-Fi literature for 2011. He is a founding member at "Forum Lacan Tel-Aviv" and member of the school of the "The International of the Forums of the Lacanian Field." Israely has published extensively with Routledge, including *Lacanian Treatment – Psychoanalysis for Clinicians* (2018), *Paradoxes in Lacanian Psychoanalysis* (2022), which was nominated by Routledge for the Gradiva Award, and *The Ethics of Lacanian Psychoanalysis* (2023). His previous works also include *The Philosophy and Psychoanalysis of Jacques Lacan* and the science fiction novel *Mesopotamia*.

Myth Psychoanalysis

Freud, Lacan and Lévi-Strauss

Yehuda Israely

Edited by
Lital Kaplan

Translated by
Mirjam Hadar

Routledge
Taylor & Francis Group
LONDON AND NEW YORK

Designed cover image: Getty Images

First published 2026
by Routledge
4 Park Square, Milton Park, Abingdon, Oxon OX14 4RN

and by Routledge
605 Third Avenue, New York, NY 10158

Routledge is an imprint of the Taylor & Francis Group, an informa business

British Library Cataloguing-in-Publication Data
A catalogue record for this book is available from the British Library

Library of Congress Cataloging-in-Publication Data
A catalog record has been requested for this book

ISBN: 978-1-041-30289-6 (hbk)
ISBN: 978-1-041-30288-9 (pbk)
ISBN: 978-1-003-77376-4 (ebk)

DOI: 10.4324/9781003773764

Typeset in Times New Roman
by Taylor & Francis Books

Contents

Introduction

Yehuda Israely

Jakobson, Lévi-Strauss, Lacan and Language

In 1942, Claude Lévi-Strauss, the anthropologist, and linguist Roman Jakobson met in New York. Both were Jewish refugees from Nazi Europe, and both had by then gained strong insights into the nature of language.

It was Jakobson to whom the secrets of language first revealed themselves. Reading Ferdinand de Saussure, he discovered that meaning evolves from arbitrary and meaningless elements, such as the sounds of a language, or its phonemes: only when these elements are combined into a word, they might yield significance. And even then, it is only when words, or "signifiers," join to make up a sentence that a context emerges in which these words gain meaning. He saw that "things" are conceptualizations arising from opposites, in the same manner as temperature is defined based on the contrast between heat and cold. Jakobson found that the most elementary opposition is that between presence and absence: cold is, in fact, nothing but the absence of heat. Any object, or feature, that doesn't seem to have an opposite "other" is therefore defined based on its presence rather than absence. The opposite of a "table," therefore, rather than being defined as a "chair" would be a non-table.

Once he defined the nature of "things," Jakobson turned to probing the mental process that charges them with meaning – and this led him to discover that "meaning" is the outcome of a comparison between "things," a comparison, that is, of pairs of opposites. Meaning is tantamount to saying about something, that it is like something else. The meaning of blue, for instance, inheres in an analogy between opposites: heat opposes cold, like red opposes blue, like emotions oppose reason. Only when we put together four elements, two pairs of opposites, between whom there is an analogy. Only then will each element gain its meaning from the context of the remaining three.

Riveted by his friend Jakobson's structural way of thinking, Lévi-Strauss put it to use when looking at phenomena he had encountered in his work as an anthropologist. Lévi-Strauss discovered that all human-cultural activity – i.e., the subject of anthropology – has a language-like structure, and that this

DOI: 10.4324/9781003773764-1

is not limited to spoken or written language alone. In the culinary domain, for instance, a dessert consisting of apple strudel served with salted caramel ice cream, involves opposites or contrasts that give distinct meaning to the combination – the pastry's crispiness is set off against the softness of the ice cream; the former's warmth contrasts with the latter's cold, while sweetness is accentuated by a salty edge. The coldness, saltiness and softness of the ice cream, in isolation, remain meaningless like isolated phonemes until they are contrasted with their opposites. The sensation of the ice-cream coldness may exist, but we couldn't call it meaningful outside a system of analogy, and analogy between contrasts. For Lévi-Strauss, the distance between illustrations deriving from the culinary domain or the arts, and tribal myths, as objects of anthropological study, was only short. These latter he interpreted by treating their core images strictly like phonemes – the in-themselves-meaningless units of sound in language – and by considering the interrelations between these as elements of the myth as well as in their context. Anthropologists of the functionalist school, before Lévi-Strauss, had treated the imagery of myth as having inherent meaning. To illustrate, think of a scholar of ancient languages who approaches a hieroglyph as though it were an icon, an image whose meaning is intrinsic. In so doing, the scholar fails to realize that the hieroglyphs constitute senseless characters, exactly like the phonemes that constitute speech, which only achieve meaning once they come together in a word.

Language consists of arbitrary elements. In the case of spoken language, these elements consist of the arbitrary vowels and consonants produced by voice and mouth. Myth's various elements, like animals, trees, stars or heavenly bodies, become arbitrarily associated with a variety of roles. So, for instance the totem, which serves as an arbitrary element representing the tribe, might be an armadillo or jaguar, but the unit of meaning composed out of arbitrary elements will be the myth, and here both armadillo and jaguar will feature. The unit of meaning consists of the relations among the totems, the relations, that is, among the different tribes represented by the totem (Lévi-Strauss 1966).

The myth about the armadillo and the jaguar who struggled until they made peace, construes the peaceful relations between one tribe whose totem is "the armadillo" and another whose totem is "the jaguar." Lévi-Strauss argued that functionalist anthropologists sought meaning in the totem only, assuming that a jaguar supports identification with an attacking force, while an armadillo suggests a defensive force. There are, similarly, approaches in psychology that believe it is possible to use ready-made lexicons to uncover the meaning of dream imagery. One example of this is the idea that a snake necessarily has phallic connotations. Lacanian psychoanalytic hermeneutics, by contrast – and like it, Lévi-Strauss's approach to mythological imagery – assumes that we cannot know anything about images in a person's dream unless we know something about their relations with other images in the dream in question.

Between the Language of Myth and the Language of the Symptom

Lévi-Strauss's discovery matched Freud's in both the depth of both men's ability to read the language of symptoms or myths, as well as their understanding and even identification with their subject of study: the mentally ill and the native. Freud came to address "the language of the mind" on learning to read the logic of hysteric symptoms by approaching them as a form of speech, a certain way of using language, with an internal logic of its own, in a way that is similar to the way in which anthropologists read and interpret myths. In the case of Anna O., for instance, he learned to "read" her symptoms in their context, finding out that Anna's paralyzed arm was the arm with which she had nursed her dying father: its paralysis communicated, among other things, feelings of guilt she had around her caring.

And here is a personal example illustrating how a symptom's meaning only emerges within context. As I was driving my car, one day, my neck suddenly cramped – just a random, physical event, it might seem. But suspecting it was a symptom – an expression of the unconscious, that is – I began to ponder the chain of thoughts that might have led up to my neck getting stuck. A few moments earlier, the radio had reported on the death of two people in a terror incident. This reminded me that earlier that morning I had heard a man I knew had died of cardiac arrest. On hearing this, I had thought he wasn't all that old and that it could happen to any one of us, without warning, just like that, out of the blue. My next thought had been that knowing we can die any moment is "like a sword above your neck." Remembering this thought led to the immediate release of my neck. So, with hindsight, this must have happened: Probably intolerable, the thought "sword above your neck" became swiftly repressed. With the fear of death repressed, the unconscious now represented the intolerable knowledge about death encapsulated in the expression "sword above your neck" in the real body rather than in consciousness. But once curiosity about the symptom led me to face my mortality again, the symptom of the cramped neck vanished (Israely 2018).

Just as in the myth's narrative, where nature and mythological animals serve as metaphors articulating the tribe's social life, we can say that the human body and the names of its organs constitute a metaphor for psychic life and its drives. Prior to Freud and Lévi-Strauss, both mental symptoms and tribal myth were inaccessible, appearing as a whole lot of unintelligible nonsense. Freud normalized the pathological and made the symptom understandable as if it were speaking in a proper language. Lévi-Strauss, from his side, may have made the greatest contribution toward questioning western cultural arrogance and superiority when he recognized the mythic logic of native peoples, and managed to decipher and interpret it for others.

Arbitrariness, Context, and Identity

It wasn't merely his sharp intellect that made Lévi-Strauss into the great interpreter of the logic of myth he was. From an early age, he reported he had not had a sense of subjectivity. He would read reality as if it were an impersonal algorithm, generating the identity of "Claude Lévi-Strauss" as a function of context, of the narrative into which he was born. He considered the idea that a person could choose who they were, a fantasy. Lacan says about this that we find ourselves in solidarity as subjects of language – whether we are natives or "savages," modern people, psychoanalysts or analysands. Any notion of autonomy, or of being self-made, is an imaginary fantasy that flies in the face of this fact.

The first domain in which Lévi-Strauss observed how language-based rules govern the life of the individual was kinship relations. Just like a word consists of letters that gain meaning only in relation to one another once they appear together in that word, humans are defined in terms of their functions within the family: father, mother, brother-in-law, daughter or son. These are all definitions that emerge based on their respective positions in relation to other members of the family: they mutually define each other. This definition by family position underlines how arbitrary reality accrues meaning only in relationships; humans are no more than "letters" in the "words" or "sentences" produced by the interrelations among family members.

At the end of World War II, Jakobson and Lévi-Strauss traveled to Paris, where they were joined by Jacques Lacan. "Infected" by the structuralist approach, Lacan took it to his revision of Freudian psychoanalysis. His statement, "the unconscious is structured like a language" reflects the idea that like language and culture, the psyche too consists of arbitrary signifiers arranged in a structure that renders them meaningful. And similar to language and culture, the psyche also operates under logical rules. For Lacan, the fact of our being desiring creatures is the outcome of our being characters in a story, driven by its plot. Our desires originate in the narratives into which we are born, and in our parents' desires, who themselves participate in the narrative. This is the source of psychoanalysis' healing potential as well as serving as the basis of one of the most important therapeutic objectives in clinical work. The more familiar a person is with the narrative in which they live, the better able they are to change it.

The Common Object of Psychoanalysis and Anthropology

This book explores the condition of the subject who-lives-in-language. This is why in this book I seek to bring to bear the perspectives of Freud, Lévi-Strauss, and Lacan, like beams casting their joint light on the same object, human life in language, from different angles, in an attempt to gain a better understanding. What is the object that psychoanalysis and structural anthropology have in common? To approach this question, we shall revert to the foundational myths Lévi-Strauss collected on his travels in the Amazonian rainforest and look at Freud's cases as mythical elements within the psychoanalytic culture.

The first common denominator consists of repressed materials and the psyche's way of dealing with them. The tribal myths of the natives are replete with regressive contents of the kind Freud identified as having become repressed in the modern adult, often leading to neurosis. These myths more or less consistently include themes associated with primary processes, whether bodily secretions or incestuous or cannibalistic relations. Regressive extra-cultural or proto-cultural images of this kind are much more transparent and exposed in native myth than in the analysand's free associations. But dreams are the exception: in them analysands, in the privileged position of not having to identify with the dream, report on regressive events in a much less censored way. They can tell themselves: That's not me, it's just my dream. Freud interprets the well-known phenomenon of the nested dream, or "dream within a dream," as a double defense against identification with the dream content.

Another point of intersection between tribal anthropology and Freudian psychoanalysis touches on something more fundamental and structural. The study group Lacan and Lévi-Strauss set up had as its joint object of interest, anthropology, psychoanalysis and the social sciences in general: art, economics, and any singularly human activity. It might be more accurate to call these "the sciences of all creatures living in language." Linguists and sociologists, anthropologists and psychoanalysts – they can all be considered not only to be using the same investigative tools, but also to be studying the same phenomenon: the way in which language structures human reality. Taken from this perspective, language, in the case of linguistics; exogamy in anthropology, and trade in economics – they all fulfil the same function, namely: exchange. Language, by allowing things to be "like" something else, enables communication between humans. The process of replacement essential to the workings of language – any language – means that we agree that the *word* X substitutes for a certain *thing*. What enables communication is the agreement people have between them about the link between the word and the meaning. In the case of trade, we trust in a coin and agree on its value, which by replacing the thing, possesses its value. Exogamous exchange relations engender peace when wives and husbands are as they were inserted into and then linked through grammatical templates. Lacan and Lévi-Strauss's study group aimed to investigate how each domain could cast light on the others.

"The way we exchange gifts among families, and brides among tribes, is the way you exchange words all the time." This is how the native people explained to Lévi-Strauss what they perceived as western people's need to talk all the time. It is through exchange that people interrelate. All social domains – kinship relations, economics, and the exchange of ideas – are rooted in language's fundamental unit of meaning, the word. Exchange occurs on the basis of an existing structure. So, for instance the structure "coin" enables changing Japanese yen into US dollars, while the "subject, object, predicate" structure makes it possible to replace words and change the meaning of a sentence. This is why Lévi-Straussian anthropology came to be known as "structural anthropology." Rather than studying cultural contents, which is the domain of ethnography, it applies itself to the language in which these contents are set down, and to the structure of this language which is reflected in the relations between its "words" and the various elements that constitute the language.

We may, for example, look at a cultural study concerning masks. The ethnographer will catalogue the different types of masks and will study the unique features of each specimen. The cultural anthropologist, by contrast, will ask: "Which elements of the mask serve as part of a language that generates meaning?" The position of the eyebrows on a Maori mask, for instance, may indicate intimidation. All cultures have their vocabulary and syntax, as well as their own definition of family membership and rules of marriage. Inter-cultural difference is expressed in different vocabularies and in the different syntactic rules of the spoken and written language, or in the rules of association in the language of kinship rules.

The affinity between structural anthropology and psychoanalysis, or between Lévi-Strauss and Lacan, has another major expression: Lévi-Strauss and Lacan agree on the importance of signifiers as pivotal, definitive elements affecting humans in a not necessarily conscious manner. And both have their doubts concerning Cartesian "thinking man" or the existentialist "choosing individual," à la Sartre. Lévi-Strauss and Lacan are "anti-essentialists" in so far as the self rather than some positivistic entity, is a meaning emerging in language. In his *The Savage Mind* (1966), Lévi-Strauss argues that whoever sticks to pre-existing and positivistic definitions of the self, organic or metaphysical, instead of realizing that the self is an outcome of language, will lose his bearings trying to explain how selves create myths when in fact they are its product, because this self, after all, is already an invention, or myth. We may reflect on the importance of such a point of departure for psychoanalysts, who find themselves confused between the ego, namely the isolated and imaginary self, and the subject, which forms a point of encounter between signifiers, a figure in a story whose desires are determined by plot.

Still, despite these influences and inspirations, there are differences between psychoanalysis and anthropology, and they must be mentioned, here, at the outset. While the anthropologist studies and describes culture, the psychoanalyst deals with a person who has a real body, who experiences pleasure and pain, and wishes to be healed. The structural anthropologist, moreover, discusses the way in which language forms the basis of culture but is not asked to explain phenomena that demonstrate the breakdown of culture, like psychosis, trauma, or sociopathy. These differences will keep showing up at various points throughout this book.

Why "The Myth of Psychoanalysis"?

The words *myth* and *psychoanalysis* interrelate in several ways that are addressed here.

The first of these is clinical: What can we, psychoanalysts, learn from structural anthropologists? What are the cultural phenomena from which we may learn something about individual-psychic processes, and what are the limits of such an exercise? Freud directly engaged with this when he compared unconscious contents in little Hans' dreams and fantasies with similar motifs in myths like that of Oedipus. Or when, in *Totem and Taboo*, he identified the inhibition of Oedipal drives as something from which the family emerges, in addition to culture. Throughout the book, we will be looking at the question of how Lévi-Strauss, especially his analysis of myth or kinship relations, may contribute to psychoanalysis and how psychoanalysts can find inspiration from, and enrich their conceptualizations by, the conceptual tools with which structural anthropologists study cultures.

Another way of connecting between psychoanalysis and myth is to ask whether psychoanalysis itself, perhaps, might be a myth, with different versions appearing in the course of history, from Freud, through Lacan, to Lévi-Strauss. Psychoanalysis, much like any other theory, is a story we tell, and it has mythical elements, *mythemes*. For Lacan, who defined four social discourses – master discourse, university discourse, hysterical discourse, and psychoanalytic discourse – the latter distinguishes itself by being conscious of its mythical nature: the remaining three discourses confuse myth and the Real. The psychoanalytic discourse manifests an awareness of the social contract that underlies its existence – resulting in a discourse that is conscious of its being purely mythical. Considering Lévi-Strauss's theory as helpful in enhancing Freud's insight, Lacan was more specific in pointing out parallel theoretical concepts between these two approaches. He expanded this thinking by defining the order of the symbolic itself as something that simultaneously connotes a person's social belonging in a culture – i.e., the domain of anthropology – and the structure of their unconscious – the realm of psychoanalysis. The name he gave to these two phenomena was "Other," with a capital O, which we may translate, with some liberty, into "the Big Other." The Big Other is the unconscious as well as culture. In the transference relations occurring in the clinic, the Big Other is associated with the analyst, in the sense that the analyst is believed to have knowledge about the patient's unconscious, as well as being a socializing agent acting on behalf of culture.

A third manifestation of the link between the two terms – myth and psychoanalysis – is that this book too is a story, adding another layer to the vast amount of already existing myths. It consists of a weave of native myths from all over the world and mythemic elements of psychoanalysis, while dwelling on Freud's paradigmatic cases: we look at Freud himself in the dream about Irma's injection; the traumas of Emma, Dora, the Rat Man, little Hans, as well as Freud's interpretation of the autobiography describing Daniel Paul Schreber's psychosis.

This book is written for a general audience that is curious about how language works in culture and in the psyche, but it is aimed primarily at therapists and analysts with a Lacanian orientation. In this book, the comparisons between analytic myths, Indigenous myths, and symptoms are a way of returning to early Lacan: to revive a textual mode of listening, to read the patient's words. There is immense clinical importance in the ability to listen to the stories in which human beings live, to read their structural logic, and in many cases to help stabilize a story that has become unsettled. This is the importance of early Lacan, and the first aim here is to illuminate these possibilities in analytic treatment; possibilities that were, in part, blurred by the development of Lacan's psychoanalysis in the direction of the Real.

This book is not only an attempt to explain how human beings exist within structures of language: myths, institutions, symptoms, and narratives, but an attempt to follow the turning point at which structure itself becomes a limit. At first, structure holds: it gives a place, a belonging, a sense, and a symbolic being. But as the clinic advances, it becomes clear that meaning, too, can become a defense, and that structure, precisely because it succeeds, may reduce being and conceal what insists beyond translation: repetition, trauma, the letter, sound, jouissance. For this reason, the movement of the book is subversive: not a replacement of one position with another, but a cut that reveals what structure enables and what it hides, and that prepares the passage from a subject who exists in language to a speaking being that is required to take responsibility for its singular knotting. In this sense, Lacan's later teaching is not an "anti-structure" that cancels what came before, but the movement in which what came before reaches its limit, where work with the Real unconscious begins.

The last chapter subverts the previous ones, as Lacan himself repeatedly did. The chapter deals with late Lacan, with the clinic of the Real. What can one say about what is, by definition, outside language? For that very reason, even here it matters to understand how the symbolic functions, if only in order to point to the Real that exceeds it. If early Lacan supports the subject who lives in the story that produces him, with desire, as a hero within a plot, late Lacan asks whether there is clinical value in going beyond the symbolic. Is there something to be gained, in analytic treatment, for a speaking being that is not limited to roles within stories?

AI was used in the preparation of this book. Chat GPT 5.2 Thinking mode was used only in chapter 12. This was done to match the tone of previous chapters, as it was added much later.

References

Israely, Y. (2018) *Lacanian Treatment – Psychoanalysis for Clinicians* (M. Hadar, Trans). Routledge.

Lévi-Strauss, C. (1966). *The Savage Mind* (English translation from the original French *Version La Pensee Savage*, 1962). University of Chicago Press.

Chapter 1

Lévi-Strauss and Structuralism

In Lévi-Strauss's basic definition, structure consists of a system characterized by mutual dependence and mutual change (1963 p. 298). Here I will try to offer an example of such a system in the linguistic domain, pointing out relations of mutual dependence and mutual change within a sentence. Let's take the following three questions: "Are you letting go of that rope?," "Are you letting go of that plan?," "Are you letting go of yourself entirely?" A change in the final words will seriously affect the meaning of "letting go," resulting in three very different meanings. "Letting go" takes on a very different meaning depending on whether it appears before "rope," a "plan," or "of oneself."

We can shift from the structure of language to that of the family: the family structure consists of a number of elements and when one of them changes, it will affect the entire family. So that when one member dies, marries, divorces, is born, and so on, all are affected. The birth of a first grandchild defines parents as grandparents, the siblings as aunts and uncles.

If we look further into structures we will see they require a more complex definition: While a structure is a type of system, conversely, for a system to qualify as a structure, more than the condition of mutual change must be met: the system also has to show a capacity for substitution and prediction. Its elements must be open to substitution, and it should be possible to foretell what will happen when the various functions are fulfilled by other elements. The structure of a sentence remains fixed even if the words of which it is made up change. It includes the unchanging functions of subject, object, and predicate. Myth is multi-layered and undergoes rewriting each time it is told or read again. One illustration is the myth of Oedipus, to which I will dedicate an entire chapter below: Lévi-Strauss's reading of this myth adds another layer to the existing versions. Sophocles' Oedipus, too, was just another such layer.

The first beginnings of the structuralist approach can be traced back to the work of the Russian ethnographer, Nikolai Sergeyevich Trubetzkoy, who founded what came to be known as Russian Formalism. His work is an example of European anthropology's ethnocentric colonialism. A genius and *wunderkind*, Trubetzkoy began his scientific studies aged 13. He was

DOI: 10.4324/9781003773764-2

fascinated by Russian folktales and took a special interest in how motifs from these tales had found their way into Finnish folklore. A Russian aristocrat and patriot, he sought to show how the wisdom of the Finnish folktales had Slavonic-Russian origins. In what sense did he resemble Lévi-Strauss? Both investigated how mythemes – myth's building blocks or units of meaning – circulate between cultures. Lévi-Strauss studied myths across the Americas. from Vancouver to the Amazon and found they included similar motifs in different variations. But Trubetzkoy, a racist, nationalist, and imperialist, wanted to show that the roots of culture were to be found in Russia, from which it then spread elsewhere. Lévi-Strauss's work does not engage in this type of search for a "first" culture, and it is shorn of any narcissistic motivation. Whether he started up north in Vancouver and moved southwards to the Amazon, or vice versa – he felt there was no "original culture" of which all the other cultures were more or less weak derivatives.

For Trubetzkoy, structuralism was based on four principles: First, the analysis shifts away from conscious to unconscious phenomena (in this he preceded Freud's reference to the conscious and unconscious). Second, the object of study, rather than elements as such, are their interrelations; in the domain of linguistics this means that the investigated phenomenon is not phonemes – the sound units of language – but rather how they come together into signifiers, i.e., units of meaning. Third, the system consists of mutually dependent elements in covariance: when one of them changes, so do the others. The fourth, and final, principle of structuralism is that it should be possible to formulate consistent rules, and by consequence to predict outcomes.

The Structuralist's Desire: Structure as Fate

What must the anthropologist or the psychoanalyst have experienced to develop the ability to consider their objects of study from a structural perspective? Or more specifically, on the strength of what desire were Lévi-Strauss, Freud, or Lacan prompted to study language – each in their respective domain – from a structural, systematic, and contextual point of view.

If we asked Lévi-Strauss, he'd answer it was a matter of humility and the belief that things carry meaning. And if we would then ask what inspired him to observe native people and their myths from an equal footing, assuming they carry meaning and follow a logic that are not inferior to western people's culture, he may well have replied that he had looked at Freud who thought of pathological and nonpathological mental activity as sharing the same psychic structure. If then, we went on to ask Freud himself who, for him, was the source of desire, informing this position of human solidarity, he would credit Charcot. Freud admired Charcot's humble, respectful attitude to his patients – which contrasted starkly with the arrogance with which he treated his medical colleagues.

Freud and Lévi-Strauss were both exceptional in the way they accepted and respected the subjects they studied without superiority. In Freud's case, he caused an uproar when he argued one did not have to be crazy to experience Oedipal urges. He believed we all have an unconscious, and participate in the psychopathology of everyday life, as well as in infantile sexuality. Freud's choice, much unlike the prevailing approach of his time, was to listen to what his patients were telling him, assuming these things could shed light on their symptoms reflected great humility.

Another aspect of Freud's modesty was his willingness to expose himself: he used his own experiences to examine the psychic structures he identified. He believed that if the Oedipus was universal, he should be able, first and foremost, to observe it in himself and in his internalized relations with his parents. He and Lévi-Strauss considered clinical and cultural superiority a defense mechanism. They both believed that this served to ensure our narcissistic pleasure by telling ourselves, that it's got nothing to do with us (Lévi-Strauss 1964). Alienation, arrogance and lack of humility are not only triggered by our fellow human's pathology, the patient, too, can take a superior attitude regarding their unconscious, claiming full control over their fate, as if unconstrained by the symbolic structures (and the unconscious mechanisms that render these structures) into which they were born.

Lévi-Strauss seems to have been "born" with a recognition that our fate is, to a considerable extent, determined by the "narrative" into which we were born, an insight more usually gained towards the end of a psychoanalysis. He had, he reported, from early on not experienced himself as having agency – i.e., as an initiating and choosing subject – but rather as being influenced and prompted into action by his surroundings and events. He was not inclined to take pride in what others might claim as their own achievement or talent. This awareness of himself as a subject emerging from a context was formative of his thinking. This was the inner structural logic at the root of Lévi-Strauss's quest after the meanings of tribal myths and it helped him refute the racist, colonialist approach dominant in university departments of anthropology. Indeed, racist politics, advanced through missionary-colonial activities, were, in Lévi-Strauss's time and well before it, propagated and backed up to no small extent by departments of anthropology.

We can learn something about how Lévi-Strauss thought of the parallel between solidarity with the native and with the neurotic patient from an experience he had, prior to his trip to Brazil, at Sainte Anne psychiatric hospital in Paris, which he had probably been invited to visit by Lacan. He interviewed a patient and later commented she had been one of the most fascinating "natives" he had ever interviewed. It was his view that he was studying human beings, whether they were psychotic or neurotic, people living in the modern west or in tribal cultures.

Lévi-Strauss's early inclination to think structurally also appears in the way in which he apprehended and processed new information. He recounts how he learned to read at the extremely young age of two, because he perceived structural elements in language. He figured out that the words *boulangerie* – bakery – and *boucherie* – butcher shop – began with a common element he managed to identify: *bou*, and he associated the sound with the written letters. Later he was to formulate this idea as the principle of repetition: the search for the stable, unchanging element in variations. Structural fate is fixed, while individual freedom occurs in the variations where the subject can choose and interpret. In the introduction to *Myth and Meaning* (1978) Lévi-Strauss mentions that he forgets what he has written once he is finished writing, and that this is probably the case because the book writes itself through him. The individual lives in myth without being aware of it and similarly, without being aware, ideas pass through Lévi-Strauss as he writes. This is how he perceives myths – in contrast with novels or history, they write themselves of their own accord.

Psychoanalysts, too, look for the motif of a dream or a symptom, without knowing its meaning. One might say that what drives the psychoanalyst, their desire, includes a structural element. The analyst's finest moment occurs when he or she identifies the recurrent expression in the patient's account and repeats it to her or him: without knowing its meaning, much like Lévi-Strauss zoomed in on – *bou.* The point of this act by the analyst is to raise to consciousness the repressed thing that is linked to the same signifier. As for the nature of the connection between the two appearances of the signifier – this the psychoanalyst leaves to the patient. An example would be a patient who draws out a particular sound when pronouncing certain words, especially rude ones. So, he may express anger at a certain person and say: "That fffffucker…." At another time he comments a certain situation "sssstinks." The interpretation will only point out the recurrence of *fffff* or *sssss*, on the assumption that these long-drawn-out consonants are signifiers. The patient's reaction reveals he has figured out the shared signified: "It's great, saying it this way" – an encounter, that is, with the pleasure or *jouissance* of it.

Lévi-Strauss, as said, treated myth as something that writes itself. This is the reason why we perceive such similarity between different myths and find, say, creation myths that repeat themselves in diverse cultures. We don't consciously initiate that kind of perception, but it is the way the mind we all share operates. This is how it works spontaneously, without the subject's conscious intention. It is, for the patient in psychoanalysis, similarly, not the point to reflect on the consciously chosen elements of their statements but to become aware of speech by way of a spontaneously emergent phenomenon, without agent. In the analytic setting, the same is also true for the therapist: the intervention emerging from her or him, too, has the quality of something that erupts spontaneously. Rather than deliberately triggering a process, the psychoanalyst rather trusts their role in the structure, which is larger than they know, and they invite the patient, too, to take this type of position.

Lévi-Strauss's Methodology: A Journey in Space and Time Between Myths

Having studied hundreds of myths, Lévi-Strauss had to somehow keep all of them in his mind simultaneously. Only in this way would he be able to observe their interrelations and figure out how a mystifying detail in one myth gains meaning from another myth originating from a geographical region at the other end of the world. Because he had to organize all these items and their links, and in the absence of the computers we have at our disposal, he stuck all this knowledge in the form of paper notes. He looked at scores of variations on the same myth, appearing across centuries-long periods. From the Amazon to Vancouver, from Patagonia to Alaska, and from 17th century Peru to myths which had changed their shape after contact with western culture.

Overwhelmed by data, Lévi-Strauss feared he might not complete his project. He knew what had happened with Saussure, the Swiss linguist, whose research, from sheer overload of data, collapsed without seeing the light of day. He worried he would lose his way in this labyrinth of myths, the endless possibilities teeming in his mind. He had already written four hefty manuscripts with analyses and interpretations of myths, but more and more variants kept presenting themselves, delaying their publication. The web of connections among the myths' shared mythemes grew ever thicker.

It was from Freud that Lévi-Strauss learned about "floating attention," and this eventually helped him with his own research. Based on the insight that culture is structured like a language, he tried to expose himself to all the signifiers that came his way and sense what struck him as worth looking at. When doing field work, he would gather information without reference to any prior pattern: this allowed him to observe unexpected things. The structural system may be either conscious or unconscious. When telling a myth, a native may be either conscious or unconscious of the meanings of its signifiers. Lévi-Strauss sought to isolate the myth's arbitrary elements – like phonemes in spoken language – and thereby to learn how to read the described events as though they were words: after all, they become meaningful through the combination of their phonemes. He acted as if he was learning a new language – a student exposed to a flow of sounds from which he would have to identify the language's meaningful sound units, and where words and syllables began and ended. Only this would enable him to get to the words' meanings.

Unlike Trubetzkoy, whose project it was to show that folktales originated in Russia in order to underpin the superiority of Russian culture, Lévi-Strauss did not believe myths could be reduced to one source. They sprang up simultaneously across the Americas, spreading every which way. Hence, for him, there was no point in trying to isolate one origin. Rather than the linear thinking espoused by Trubetzkoy and others, Lévi-Strauss's approach was rhizomatic. A typical rhizomatic structure is that of grass, which rather than developing vertically, grows laterally or sideways. While trees for instance grow in a very distinct, upward direction: roots – stem – branches – leaves/fruit, the rhizome's roots interconnect laterally. There is no linear hierarchy in the rhizome, and each bit of root may connect to any other bit of root. The fig tree behaves like this too: its aerial roots both interlink and connect to the tree trunk from which they sprout. Something like this can be said about myths: you can pinpoint neither first nor last. This, too, was how Lévi-Strauss thought of tribal modes of exchange or influence. He believed it was why myths tended to be so basically similar – provided, that is, we can look through their variants. Since myths are rhizomatically related, the choice of one myth as a starting point while considering other myths as variants is rather arbitrary. When dealing with particularly inaccessible parts of a myth, Lévi-Strauss would first look at communities in the close vicinity, but if this did not yield an explanation, he would turn to communities further afield.

Still, given the linear, sequential nature of writing and speech, Lévi-Strauss had to start with one myth in order then to map its connections to others. The myth he selected for that purpose was about the origins of the fire used for roasting meat (Lévi-Strauss 1964), and he described adjacent myths as variants. He studied them from a *synchronic* perspective: how does a myth change shape while preserving its idea across geographic distances. He also considered them *diachronically*, namely how a myth in one geographic location changes over time. When we place concepts sequentially, we put them in diachronic order, and when, by contrast, we arrange them, say, like patches of different colors simultaneously observed on a canvas, the ordering principle is synchronic. To return to my above description of the principles of structuralism, Lévi-Strauss saw myth as a matrix of all possible combinations of mythemes within a consistent structure. Myth is the source of information from which linear stories can be construed. That a narrative will take the shape of one particular word following another reflects the fact that despite the rhizomatic nature of our perception, we must, for the sake of communication – as speech and listening occur on the temporal axis – arrange it in linear sequence. We give our knowledge about the world the shape of stories. Prior to the invention of writing, information had to be presented in linear fashion due to the constraints of spoken language, with words following each other in sequence. Since we cannot say more than one word at a time, concepts must appear in a sequence following the order of speech.

One illustration of information organized narratively, or diachronically in a process unfolding along the axis of time, even though it aims to render an a-temporal principle, is the following: Plagued by a cruel southerly wind, the Vancouver natives could not go out to sea. Then the fishermen turned to the skate fish, which is black on top and white underneath. They asked the skate to intervene on their behalf with the southerly wind. After long, arduous negotiations, the skate managed to persuade the wind to settle. It would blow one day and abstain the other.

This narrative is an expression of the principle of the binary. But it is presented in the form of a story that unfolds over time: first the natives addressed the fish; next the fish turned to the southerly wind. But what we really have here is information about the nature and workings of a principle.

And here is a clinical illustration to show how useful it is to extract the principle a narrative represents. A patient says he has a fear, perhaps irrational, that once everything in his life will be all right – work, his relations with his partner, the children – cancer is sure to present itself. This is a narrative form of Freud's pleasure principle: absolute pleasure equals the absence of tension, homeostasis, nirvana, or, in other words: death. The patient fears the narrative effects of the formula, as if the latter took place on the axis of time and will at some point catch up with him. There is no real danger of nirvana breaking out once things at work settle down, but the wish for absolute peace equals the death drive.

The Myth about the Origin of the Cold

The myth about the origin of the cold which we shall now consider offers a good example of how Lévi-Strauss analyzed geographic links between myths to find their meaning. In the wake of a spell of extreme cold, the shaman of a Peruvian tribe declared the following three groups of tribe members to be guilty: twins, those who were born with a harelip, and those were delivered bottom or feet first, in a breech birth. They had to atone for their sins to save the rest of the tribe. When Lévi-Strauss read this myth, he wondered about the connection: why exactly these three groups? In search of a clue, he went on reading other myths in hopes they would help him understand. In another Peruvian myth, a woman became pregnant from a man who pretended to be her husband. Upon discovering she was pregnant, she rushed to have intercourse with her husband. The myth tells that the twins who were born were the offspring of two fathers, and like their fathers, one was born good, and the other sly. In another myth, from Vancouver, two sisters were given false promises of marriage, leading to the birth out of wedlock of two cousins. Even though these two boys were cousins rather than twins, they are a variation on the mytheme of a pair of fraudulently begotten children. If we look at the Peruvian myth's reference to harelips, it seems to pick up the Vancouver myth: when a rabbit peeped at the sexual parts of one of the sisters who gave birth out of wedlock, it was punished by being hit on the nose, leading to the hare's cleft upper lip. The third feature – that of the breech birth – derives from another myth: This myth recounts a case of sibling rivalry, with the twin brothers struggling for the right of primogeniture. It is the brother who is in the greatest rush to be first, who is born feet first. This myth about the twin brothers, Lévi-Strauss (1978) found among the Tupinamba tribe, from the Atlantic coast of Brazil.

This is one example of the methodology Lévi-Strauss used to map a myth. The mythemes "deception," "peeping," and "stealing the right of primogeniture" – or "rivalry in the family" – are variations on the breaking of a taboo. The more abstract mytheme is the principle of splitting: twins in the womb, two fathers – one each for each child – and the splitting of the hare's lip which initiates a splitting of the entire body. All this imagery shares the concept of splitting, and it runs through all three narratives. What, then, is the shaman's message to his community if we translate it into the language of logic? The reason for the cold spell lies in division, a split among the group members. And those whose role, in the myth, symbolizes splitting will have to make amends for the taboo's breach. They will have to heal division. Had Lévi-Strauss not studied myths from the farthest corners of the Americas, the shaman's instructions would have remained incomprehensible.

Lévi-Strauss constructs the story of the myth out of a whole lot of other myths, rites and rituals, and like him, the psychoanalyst makes sense of the patient by looking at symptoms, dreams, and other expressions of the unconscious. And just like in anthropology these symbols or signifiers will derive from a variety of places, something like this must be the case with the analysand. In psychoanalysis we do something similar when we shift attention to another domain of the patient's life seeking to find meaning for what remains unintelligible in the original context. For example, a patient was obsessively preoccupied with the thought her husband was cheating. In the absence of any indications, it was a riddle why she was so obsessed. At the same time, she had a sexual fantasy about a man and two women. The fantasy, then, casts light on why she carries the obsessive thought; What probably happens in the unconscious is that she produces the fantasy for pleasure but without awareness that that is the reason for keeping this thought in her mind. When she interprets to herself why this thought of another woman is on her mind, she assumes that its because she is afraid it will happen. This way she is unaware that she herself is producing it, and this is the source of her jealousy. Jealousy, then, takes a ride on the pleasure she takes in her fantasy.

Influences on Lévi-Strauss

Like the myths he studied, Lévi-Strauss's own theory, too, emerged from many different influences. It was not just his natural way of thinking that led him to his insights. He was inspired by the work of many others, not just Freud and Jakobson.

Franz Boas, Margaret Mead, and Post-Colonialism

Franz Boas, an American anthropologist of German-Jewish origins, was open about his envy of linguists. Lévi-Strauss met Boas, among the most prominent of US anthropologists of his time, when he arrived in New York as a refugee in 1939. Until then he had been mainly exposed to European colonialist influences. Boas, more than once, mentioned to his student Lévi-Strauss how he envied linguists for their discipline's structural nature. Such comments may have sharpened Lévi-Strauss's attention when, later on, he encountered Jakobson.

Boas upheld an ethics that honored pluralism and difference. While criticizing ethnocentrism and racism, he did not, like Lévi-Strauss, look for the universal rules under which all human beings are equal, or for solidarity in language. His object of study was the singularity of specific cultures. Boas's tendency was towards the ethnographic more than anthropological. His inquiry was aimed less toward the essence of human society and more toward the particularity of specific societies. Nevertheless, we may say he helped Lévi-Strauss formulate his question: what can we, as anthropologists, learn from linguists?

Margaret Mead was one of Boas's star students, and like Lévi-Strauss, she too was strongly influenced by Freud. Psychoanalysis, said Freud in "Civilization and its Discontents" (1961), seeks to heal the damage done by civilization. Mead turned western racism upside down. Taking a liberal perspective, she interpreted Freud's position as western puritanism while idealizing Samoa's native culture. From her research in Samoa, she concluded that members of native cultures are sexually much freer, having to struggle with less sexual frustrations and their fallout. Lacan disagreed with this interpretation of Freud. Freud, he argued, had been thinking of all language-using creatures, which is to say that the sickness from which we suffer is language as such – and not western language alone. Every speaking being, who lives within language, and uses phonemes and signifiers, is cursed and cast out of the paradise of non-mediated reality. Humans dwell no longer in the Real and have to make do with symbolic substitutes. This is the damage done by civilization.

Durkheim and the Social Collective

In his sociological investigations, Durkheim reached the conclusion that "Protestants commit more suicide than Catholics." Over and beyond the individual component in someone's wish to put an end to their life, may there be a more specific cultural effect involved in their choice? This was one of the research questions Emile Durkeim formulated. The first to define a social phenomenon as a scientific object, Durkheim is considered the founder of modern sociology.

The approach to the collective as a type of creature was initiated by Durkheim and transferred into anthropology by his admiring nephew, Marcel Mauss. All this formed the background to Lévi-Strauss's eventual insight that the totem functioned as signifier of the collective. He understood that, like in Durkheim's approach, natives, too, treat the collective as an entity. This helped him decipher kinship relations and myths, and how they suggest the interrelations constituting the collective.

Marcel Mauss – Social Order and the Individual Unconscious as the Great Other

Mauss had a great impact on Lévi-Strauss. It is from him that he took the idea of unconscious forces determining people's social-cultural behavior. But Mauss seems to have left his marks on Lévi-Strauss emotionally too, communicating his passion. That passion took the shape of a wish to analyze cultural phenomena with the tools and exactitude of linguists. Structuralism, as such, emerged in response to this desire. Lévi-Strauss wrote the introduction to Mauss's seminal *The Gift*, he learned from him, and eventually eclipsed him.

Mauss believed that unconscious desires, whose expressions Freud identified in slips of the tongue, symptoms, and dreams, are how the collective effects individuals, who – nevertheless – perceive themselves free of unconscious social influence. It was in this spirit that Lévi-Strauss analyzed the behaviors of native people, without expecting them to be necessarily aware of their role in the structure. Picking up this line of thought, Lacan defined language as the point of intersection between unconscious desires and the social order behind them. He created the notion of the "big other" or "the Other" which he related to both language as the collective domain, and the personal unconscious.

At a later point, Lacan added into this equation the psychoanalyst's position in the transference: The psychoanalyst is the Other in the sense of being ascribed knowledge about the patient's unconscious. Thus, in the psychoanalyst the internal unconscious and the external social collective come together. The psychoanalyst in the clinic represents the authority collective norms have vested in her or him; at the same time, the analyst is believed to have knowledge about the unconscious of the patient who says to himself: "You probably know better than I what's going on in my mind." The Other is the unconscious by way of an internal language system guiding the subject's actions without the latter's awareness, but at the same time it constitutes the vocabulary the subject owns: the dictionary to which the subject, and not they alone, is exposed. This is the symbolic Other – not the Imaginary other who will be a certain persona, usually attributed parental or divine qualities.

De Saussure – On the Arbitrary and the Ability to Stop

Ferdinand de Saussure, the Swiss linguist, is responsible for highlighting the arbitrariness that became key to Lévi-Strauss's approach to research. For Saussure, the signifier is arbitrary – in contrast with onomatopoeia, where representation resembles the thing represented. The word *fizz*, for example, corresponds to the sound it represents – bubbling or frothing; the word *clink* reproduces the sound of glass ringing against glass. But these cases, and onomatopoeia as a whole, are rare. They really are the exception that proves the rule: The arbitrary signifier does not derive meaning from its sound, but from a context formed by other arbitrary signifiers. This approach enabled Lévi-Strauss not to be distracted: whether the tribes were represented by either the armadillo or the jaguar totem was wholly unrelated to their actual possession of shields or claws. The totems' meaning is inherent in their joint appearance in a myth in which two tribes make peace: the myth settles the groups' interrelations in this manner. The jaguar might have been substituted by a tapir – as long as it makes peace with the totem of the other tribe. In Saussure, we might say, we can identify the beginnings of contextuality in Lacan's sense. But Lacan is more radical and severs signifier from object. The signifier does not represent the object – it creates the signified. Meaning inheres not in the signified, but in the signifier.

Another way in which Saussure was a source of inspiration for Lévi-Strauss, involved the latter's awareness of the former's failure, something I mentioned earlier. It was said about Saussure that he was so bent on mapping everything that he got lost in the details and never published his magnum opus. Lévi-Strauss's nightmare was of meeting a similar fate. At some stage during his research, he realized he had to stop collecting data and start organizing and summarizing them. The result was four thick tomes, the *Mythologies*, bringing together thousands of key mythemes. Lévi-Strauss could well have continued collecting myths, analyzing and compiling many more such volumes. For us psychoanalysts, the idea of imposing a halt or caesura is important too. A patient may talk ad infinitum, moving between myths, mythemes, and signifiers, and it is up to us, psychoanalysts, to bring this to a halt and cut the session, or, alternatively, to interpret one idea suggested by the patient's dream while foregoing others.

References

Freud, S. (1961). Civilization and its discontents (J. Strachey, Trans.). In *The standard edition of the complete works of Sigmund Freud* (Vol. 21, pp. 64–145). London: Hogarth Press.

Lévi-Strauss, C. (1963). *Structural anthropology* (C. Jacobson & B. G. Schoepf, Trans.). Basic Books.

Lévi-Strauss, C. (1964). *The raw and the cooked* (J. Weightman & D. Weightman, Trans.). University of Chicago Press.

Lévi-Strauss, C. (1978). *Myth and meaning*. (J. E. Hochberg, Trans.). London: Routledge & Kegan Paul.

Lévi-Strauss, C. (1987). *Introduction to the work of Marcel Mauss* (F. Baker, Trans.). Routledge & Kegan Paul. The University of Chicago Press.

Chapter 2

The Myth of the Subject's Creation in the Encounter with the Signifier

Yehuda Israely

This book aims to cast some light on the Real. While the Real cannot be wholly clarified, it can to some extent. Various disciplines have attempted this through their different theoretical lenses, guided by Freud, Lévi-Strauss, or Lacan. The present effort is to bundle together the different rays they have cast, even though it is fated – like all attempts to capture the Real – to be yet another among many mythic accounts, like the proverbial invisible person, whose shape we can only guess from behind its cloak. The Real shimmers through the Amazonian myths about animals in the jungle, in patients' talk when they visit the clinic, as well as in psychoanalysts' theorizing.

Psychoanalysis, of course, is not exempted from the rules of symbolic structuring and mythologization. In psychoanalysis as myth, and in theoreticians' efforts to produce myths of psychic life, the birth of the subject plays a key role. The myth of the subject's birth seeks to capture something real about the emergence of human beings.

How can we catch a glimpse of the Real in relation to the subject's birth? Lévi-Strauss believed that structure – basic, shared and foundational to so many aspects of human, cultural life – came closest to the Real. For Lacan, by contrast, it was the body's pleasure or *jouissance* that most closely approached it. This is exactly where he set himself apart from Lévi-Strauss – who focused on communities rather than on the physical, embodied organism. Unlike Lacan and Lévi-Strauss, for Freud the drive, on the seam between Symbolic and Real, between body and mind, approaches the Real most closely. We will start recounting the story of the subject's genesis with him.

The Drives According to Freud

The metaphor Freud chose for the human drive is that of the steam engine. Like the steam engine, the drive involves source, pressure, and release. Lacan, after Freud, formulated the mind's action in terms of cybernetic processes of meaning making, or of a computer. In Freudian terms, anger is "released," whereas in Lacanian ones we "construct an anger-arousing story." The implication is that a person who releases their anger actually produces it in doing so.

DOI: 10.4324/9781003773764-3

What caused Freud to use the steam engine metaphor? Unlike instinct, the drive is a "literary creation." It results from the encounter between our being instinctual creatures, on the one hand, and belonging in language, on the other. The steam engine metaphor which Freud used to describe the drives, derives from the domain of physics and is associated with the industrial revolution. When we make sense of a metaphor the signifier introduces an additional signified. When we choose a metaphor like "strong like a lion" or "strong like a rock," we may also suggest: "wild like a lion" and "impervious like a rock." So, what does the metaphor tell us about the nature of the drive? A steam engine is manmade, not a natural object. It is the product of human invention and technology. The psychic drive, too, is manmade, in contrast with biological instinct. While instinct fulfils a genetically encoded need, drive looks for semantically determined pleasure.

One feature of biological need is that, once it is satisfied, a drop in the level of inner impulse can be registered, but Freud observed that this is not the case with the drives. In "Beyond the Pleasure Principle" (1920) Freud looks at the mystery of why non-satisfaction is a source of attraction. Why do people seek to repeat stressful situations? Is there basic masochism behind human dissatisfaction? Lacan's answer is: Yes! This is what we're like, and language is to blame. Being a replacement for the Real, language always lacks actuality. At the same time language also offers humans something the Real cannot provide. What comes into being following the "first death" survives the second: in substituting for the thing itself, the symbol survives the organism's death. Through language and symbols, the subject can identify with what goes beyond their organic existence, staking out their future through heritage and tradition. Language is not limited to the speech or writing the subject uses but also embraces the language-based cultural systems in which the subject participates. And, in addition, language covers the social syntax of family relations, a country's laws, and the titles a subject carries among their fellow subjects. Language enables us to belong and participate in a structure. This structure consists of a story or narrative through which the human organism dynamically emerges. While the structure acts upon, and drives, the subject, the surrounding world regards the subject as someone who makes choices, and so the subject learns to regard itself as someone who makes choices. When a child says something surprising or clever, people laugh, and this makes her repeat it. The child had no intention to amuse but the amused response makes the child feel that he is attributed with the intention to make them laugh. It's now that the intention has entered the situation, merely because he believes, and he is probably right. This is how they produced a subject.

If we look beyond the organism that sustains the subject, we may say that the entry into language inaugurates a creature whom we may consider having intentionality – or in other words, a "soul." Through their actions, in the course of their lives, people make a "name" for themselves, and this name survives, even after they die. In native cultures, the dead stay part of the community by virtue of the group's common belonging to the totem. Jewish tombstones carry the following text: "May his or her soul be bound up in the bonds of life."

As mentioned, for Freud (1905) the drive has an origin, an impulse, an aim, and an object. The origin is an internal, physical stimulus, which occurs in some parts of the body and has a conscious representation. Let's say, a rumbling stomach. The impulse is the force exerted to stimulate action, which, in its turn, aims to satisfy the need. The urge or drive persists; organic satisfaction does not always appease psychic hunger. Though the aim of the drive is satisfaction – satisfaction of what is another question. Not quite of the need, since eating doesn't stop once the stomach is full. The subject is not hungry for food: they hunger for meaning and cannot get satisfaction in the domain of the actual – where the drive, however, is expressed. We understand that an actual full stomach will never meet the need for emotional security – which can however be satisfied by verbally conducted communication. To illustrate, Lacan refers to what happens when we order food in a restaurant: here it is not simply eating the food itself that is responsible for satisfaction, but rather the conversation about the various dishes on offer. This is also a reason for the current popularity of food shows on TV, where the audience don't come near tasting the actual food. Rather than the thing itself, the drive is directed at the signifier or meaning.

Drive and the Creation of the Subject According to Lacan

For Freud, the positivist, psychic reality is a priori, given, as though its existence needs no explanation. Since for Lacan, the postmodernist, psychic reality is not given, it may crumble, like in the case of psychosis, unlike Freud for whom the status of psychic reality is not subverted under psychosis. Freud searches for meaning in Schreber's delusions while Lacan sees them as the result of the fragmentation of the symbolic order.

As Lacan sees it, mental reality, and hence the manner in which the individual constructs external reality, results from the interweaving of three registers or orders: the Symbolic, the Imaginary, and the Real. The foundation of the subject requires a constructive process, and this is achieved by entering language. The object's function in this process is to be lost, or to come up short, generating an absence around which the subject germinates. The object may take the shape of the breast from which the baby is weaned, or of sexual difference suggesting that something is or might be missing. The foundation of the subject consists of replacing object by signifier. One instance is how the first-born child's earlier claim on attention when a little sibling is born is compensated and substituted by the title of "eldest" or "big boy."

Lacan conceives of the object as the thing being "orbited" in the ballistic sense: rather than being taken hold of it is encircled or surrounded. There is another sense, too, in which the object orbits the subject through subterfuge:

it promises satisfaction only to offer the signifier instead, by way of a replacement. This trick works by holding out the temptation an already-lost object can be retrieved: its absence is what prompts the action from the outset. The subject comes into being around the scar left by the lost object, or: the subject is defined as one who has no object. She or he clings to the signifier that substitutes the object, the same signifier that represents them as they enter the language-based community. One cannot be part of a family unless one functions as the son or daughter of someone else, or in any other such familial role. And, clinging to the signifier to partake in the myth, the subject becomes a desiring subject. This is for two reasons: they lack an object, and, in addition, now there are signifiers onto which they can latch their hope for satisfaction.

In the symbolic structure, the subject is reciprocally constituted with a view to other signifiers representing other things in the world. Absence and signifier join and produce desire, and this the subject experiences as vitality. Attributing this sense of vitality to the signifiers around them, natives and young children will tend to think animistically, while once they "enter into language" they will transform into "intending" subjects. The analogical structure that produces meaning by obeying the statement "A stands to B as C stands to D" supports an animistic frame of mind: inanimate objects, here, exist in language much like the self: if I live in language, and the object is in language, too, it follows that the object lives. In the course of their education into the rational thinking that replaces mythical thinking, children must "kill" a considerable part of their surrounding world. Under the sway of reason, the similarity between things rendered by the word "like" does not suffice to make them come to life. We shall further investigate this in the chapter dedicated to animism.

Lacan's Big Bang Myth

To describe the subject's emergence as a result of loss of the object and its substitution by the signifier, Lacan invented a version of the creation myth which he presented in the form of the graph of desire during his 1957–1958 seminar on the formations of the unconscious. Once upon a time, in a different logical temporality and hypothetical reality, the perfect subject and the perfect Other coexisted as one body. In fact, designating them as such misleadingly presupposes an act of division, but we can say with hindsight that, sometime in the past, these two were "in this thing" which had yet to undergo separation. And this is when the big bang occurred. Perfect subject and perfect Other collapsed into each other, much like particles in a particle accelerator, and once the smoke rose, there were three elements: the absent Other, the split subject, and the residual object *a*. The Other equals the symbolic order, language and culture, which may be represented by a parent or any other authority figure invested with the law. The symbolic order is imperfect: it neither formulates nor expresses everything. Hence, in their role as the Other a parent cannot but disappoint and reveal themselves as lacking.

Both Other and subject now suffer lack as a result of losing the object that connected them. Lacan calls this linking object "l'objet petit *a*" – the object with a small a. But we mustn't forget this is a myth: the perfect subject is an oxymoron. Language does not cover all of being, and the subject right from the start is grounded in the lack the word creates within the organism. Neither subject nor Other were ever perfect, and the same is true for the space they shared, which went lost in the act of separation: the lost residue, or object *a*. It too was attributed presence in retrospect, in light of its loss. Only after the event was it invested with concrete form – like the nipple from which the baby was weaned. This myth underlines the idea that perfection comes to grief not only in the subject but also in the Other. In the narrative of infant and mother, not only does the infant lose the nipple, but so does the mother. In this scene of separation, the mother too ends up being castrated.

We can trace Lacan's myth of the subject's creation in the autobiography of Helen Keller, in her description of her encounter with language. Here the broken pieces of her doll function as object *a*, the missing object that spells entry to the signifier.

Helen Keller's Birth as a Subject

In our encounter with language, we are born as subjects. For the pre-verbal infant, every four-legged animal is a "woof woof." It takes time for infants to slice up the world into distinct objects by using different signifiers such as "miaow miaow" or "bah bah." But who can report back on this moment of our emergence? Can people testify to the moment they are born as participants in the conversation? Can they point at the moment when they became individuals who divide the world into objects by means of signifiers? Australian aboriginals express this when they say that if they cannot recount their mythology, which they call "dream time," the world will stop existing. This, though, is myth rather than actual memory.

Maybe we should be asking an even more fundamental question: Is there anyone who can describe their own experience of how language infused them and the world with life, and how without it, everything, them and the world, would be dead?

There is only one person in the history of mankind who was present at their own birth as a subject and able to bear witness to it. In her book *The Story of my Life* (Keller 1903) Helen Keller describes this moment. Her high intelligence, in combination with her low communicational ability due to early onset deafness and blindness, made for the unusual circumstances that enabled her to experience, and subsequently recounted how she was a mere organism until she was able to enter the human, symbolic narrative.

> One day, while I was playing with my new doll, Miss Sullivan put my big rag doll into my lap also, spelled "*d-o-l-l*" and tried to make me

> understand that "*d-o-l-l*" applied to both. Earlier in the day we had had a tussle over the words "*m-u-g*" and "*w-a-t-e-r*." Miss Sullivan had tried to impress it upon me that "*m-u-g*" is mug and that "*w-a-t-e-r*" is water, but I persisted in confounding the two. In despair she had dropped the subject for the time, only to renew it at the first opportunity. I became impatient at her repeated attempts and, seizing the new doll, I dashed it upon the floor. I was keenly delighted when I felt the fragments of the broken doll at my feet. Neither sorrow nor regret followed my passionate outburst. I had not loved the doll. In the still, dark world in which I lived there was no strong sentiment or tenderness. I felt my teacher sweep the fragments to one side of the hearth, and I had a sense of satisfaction that the cause of my discomfort was removed. She brought me my hat, and I knew I was going out into the warm sunshine. This thought, if a wordless sensation may be called a thought, made me hop and skip with pleasure.
>
> We walked down the path to the well-house, attracted by the fragrance of the honeysuckle with which it was covered. Someone was drawing water and my teacher placed my hand under the spout. As the cool stream gushed over one hand she spelled into the other the word *water*, first slowly, then rapidly. I stood still; my whole attention fixed upon the motions of her fingers. Suddenly I felt a misty consciousness as of something forgotten, a thrill of returning thought; and somehow the mystery of language was revealed to me. I knew then that "*w-a-t-e-r*" meant the wonderful cool something that was flowing over my hand. That living word awakened my soul, gave it light, hope, joy, set it free! There were barriers still, it is true, but barriers that could in time be swept away.
>
> I left the well-house eager to learn. Everything had a name, and each name gave birth to a new thought. As we returned to the house every object which I touched seemed to quiver with life. That was because I saw everything with the strange, new sight that had come to me. On entering the door I remembered the doll I had broken. I felt my way to the hearth and picked up the pieces. I tried vainly to put them together. Then my eyes filled with tears; for I realized what I had done, and for the first time I felt repentance and sorrow. I learned a great many new words that day. I do not remember what they all were; but I do know that *mother, father, sister, teacher* were among them, words that were to make the world blossom for me, "like Aaron's rod, with flowers." It would have been difficult to find a happier child than I was as I lay in my crib at the close of that eventful day and lived over the joys it had brought me, and for the first time longed for a new day to come.
>
> (Keller 1903 pp. 22–24).

Before taking a closer look at Helen Keller's description of her birth-as-subject, this is the place to go back to three of Lacan's earlier mentioned structural definitions of the subject of the unconscious: 1. the intentional subject is one whose existence we assume; 2. the subject is one who yearns due to object loss, and 3. the subject is one who is represented by a signifier which is part of a web of other signifiers and subjects.

How do we understand Helen Keller's account? As long as she had a hard time learning the words her teacher was trying to impart, and would erupt into a rage, throwing and breaking things, followed by a sense of indifference, she was in a primitive state, reminiscent of myth's primeval world. That world offers two options: either a retentive withdrawal, a constipative state from which nothing is issued; or an explosive eruption, where in the absence of any restraint, the difference between inside and out collapses.

What happens next in Keller's account is her encounter with structure. Anne Sullivan, her teacher, tried to teach Keller the concept of "doll" by associating the spelling: d-o-l-l with the two dolls. She also tried to get across that j-u-g is unlike w-a-t-e-r on grounds of the divergence in both their tactile experience and imprinted spelling. This follows the same logic as what led the young Lévi-Strauss – in the personal myth of creation I mentioned in Chapter 1 – to understand language through its structural qualities, when he figured out that the initial characters *Bou* occur in both *Boucherie* and *Boulangerie*. It is hard to tell whether Helen learned anything at this early stage; she mainly describes her own impatience with her teacher's attempts. These attempts, however, clearly form the backdrop to the moment of insight, which was soon to follow, once she understood language. From this moment on, everything that carried a name turned into an object with a life of its own. The regret Keller later felt about the loss of her doll was related to the fact that the doll, too, had suddenly become a living creature, in the animistic sense of owning intentionality. Attributing life is the outcome of attributing intentionality: since all these objects, much like herself, have a name in language, they must – also like herself – have a will.

Helen would not have been able to emerge as a subject had she not broken her doll. The cognition tying together the sense of water and the impression of signifiers her teacher left on her hand would not have done the job. Had she not experienced the loss of the doll, the potential of lack, expressed through the substitution signifier-for-thing, or symbol-for-real, would not have occurred.

Helen Keller entered the world as a subject once she began to experience herself as an intentional agent – even if, in this case, the intention was destructive. Guilt is a necessary corollary of emergent subjectivity as an intentional agent. A patient with a psychotic structure – one in which the subject is not fully present – once told me how he wished he could feel guilt for what he did, just the way subjects who experience themselves as intending agents must feel. He, instead, felt himself part of a cosmic plan over which he had no control and in which he was only trying to figure out his own role. The unconscious deploys guilt as a signifier of subjectivity. It is therefore not surprising that in most creation myths, across most cultures, the entry into civilization comes with a sense of sin and guilt, as in the case of Prometheus stealing the fire from the gods, or of Adam and Eve who become cultural creatures only after covering their nakedness following their transgression. Exile from paradise, and its attendant shame and guilt, are all indispensable to the emergence of culture.

Once the object (the doll) was lost, and she encountered the signifier (the feel of water and of the spelled word w-a-t-e-r; and subsequently becoming aware of the spelling of the word d-o-l-l), Helen was overwhelmed by desire for the world around her. Once the signifier enabled events-in-the-world to turn into objects, she could feel her desire as subject, an experience based on the absent object. To make this more accessible: imagine you participate in a conference where you can present yourself only by wearing a name tag, and you are allowed to address others solely by using the label they, too, are wearing. The conference stands for the world, and the name label stands for the signifier. Helen Keller found herself outside the world, having no signifiers and no ability to communicate. Her moment of revelation occurred when she, too, understood the principle of the signifier, adopted it, and began "wearing" it, an entry ticket to the world of things represented in language.

Now that the subject's life-giving desire had sparked, she immediately began to perceive the surrounding world in that way: quivering with life. Everything she could name she now infused with life. Water too sprang to life in this moment. Signifiers mark the world's objects, tying them together into a web, and into a narrative in which they operate, and in which they have intentionality and are animated. As soon as we name something, we invite it into the community of speakers and treat it like a desiring subject – for he or she, too, are touched by language. Only later in life does this experience come to a halt under the sway of an approach that is considered rational. Remnants of this we can, for example, see in the language of builders who say about the dry concrete that "it thirsts for water."

The Link Between Sign and Signifier – Our Senses Can Perceive Neither God nor Love

While a sign represents a thing and derives its meaning from it, the signifier represents meaning deriving from the relations among signifiers, regardless of whether it has an actual object. In her writings, Helen Keller explained how her understanding of language evolved beyond the first relationship between the sign impressed on her hand and water, as well as the sense of the cold flow touching her skin. She understood the function of the signifier. Much later she was asked how she understood the meaning of the things she read if she experienced neither vision nor sound and had to make do with words only. How did she know what the moon was if she had never seen it? She answered that neither God nor love are subject to sense perception. Love is a concept. She understood signifiers through their interrelations with other signifiers. In fact, her personal experience corroborates Jakobson, Lévi-Strauss, and

Lacan's arguments concerning signifiers gaining meaning from other signifiers. It is through being embedded in their context, that signifiers determine the signified – i.e., meaning; signifiers, unlike signs, are not tethered to things. Helen Keller never saw the moon, but if she would read the braille dictionary entry for it, or for the notion of love, she would encounter more signifiers, and if she would then look them up too, and so on, covering the entire dictionary, then all these signifiers would act to support each other's meanings – without her having any contact with the actual world. Arguably, Helen Keller had to feel the actual water in order then to associate it with the signifier; arguably, the link between the signifier, communicated by touch, and the wet, cool thing constitutes the point of contact between lexicon and real world, but the connection, rather than being between two elements, is quadruple. The link between signifier and thing is valid by force of comparing two signifier-signified pairs: the signifier "water" stands to the cool, wet thing, as the signifier "doll" stands to the broken doll on the ground. It is therefore the *relationship* between these two signifiers that offers a first grounding for analogy, for meaning – even before departing the lexicon and entering the world.

Lacan illustrates the non-essential foundation of the signifier, i.e., the absence, in it, of a thing, by pointing at the drives. In his discussion he focuses on four drives in a two-by-two matrix: the oral and anal drives, voice and gaze. One division into pairs is between drives associated with the mouth: orality, and voice, and those associated with authority: the gaze overseeing anal-cultural behaviors. Lacan assumes that the drives, rather than being based in actual reality, are symbolic. The concrete object is an unnecessary addition. Beyond her experience of the link between sign and sensation – in the case, for instance, of the water, Helen Keller's testimony relating to God or love, shows that no object is required to imbue the signifier with meaning. This confirms Lacan and Lévi-Strauss's structuralist approach. It is not from the thing itself that the signifier receives meaning but from the relations between it and other signifiers, and rather than rendering an object it represents the subject who enounces it. The signifier creates the object by construing it.

Object Loss, Sacrifice, and Divination

The Polynesian shaman would stretch the membrane surrounding the entrails of a sacrificial pig dedicated to women giving birth and hold it up against the sunlight. The spirit of the totem addressed him through the membrane's white webbing. It told him about the future health and well-being of mother and newborn. Haruspicy, the art of reading the future from the entrails of a sacrificial animal, is an archaic ritual found in cultures across the world. Like Helen Keller's doll, the sacrificial animal must die in order to be substituted by a meaningful text.

Even though the "text," in the case of reading the entrails of the dead pig, is not yet alphabetic, or even hieroglyphic, we can definitely identify communication with spirits or gods who are perceived to have subjectivity and with whom there is enough common ground for exchange. They are said to communicate messages we might want to define as "proto-texts," and it is the role of the shaman to decipher these. This suggests a similarity between shaman and psychoanalyst who are both in the business of deciphering, something Lacan discusses in his 18th seminar (1970–1971), when he mentions the ancient Chinese technique of predicting the future by interpreting the cracks appearing on a tortoise shell when heated. Here the two types of reading – of signs and of text – come together in the fact that the Chinese fortune tellers engraved their interpretation of the signs on the same shell. This written text amounts to a translation of the signs formed by the cracks, supporting the assumption of there being a text requiring translation. This is what the psychoanalyst does with their patient's talk. When the patient recounts a dream and the psychoanalyst finds meanings and intentions in it, she helps the patient believe that there "is" someone there. This is how the psychoanalyst interprets expressions of the unconscious in the dream, the symptom and other formations. The shaman assumes the presence of intentionality – whether it is that of a god or a devil – and similarly the psychoanalyst postulates an unconscious, intending subject. And much like the signs on the tortoise shell, or the sacrificial animal's entrails are translated into a "text," symptoms are translated into an "interpretation" of the form: "Your unconscious is telling us that…." The Freudian unconscious is neither more nor less mythic than any god or devil in whose existence the shaman believes.

The emergence of the subject through the loss of the object can be observed in various myths describing the birth of the subject – whether in the personal or the social sense. The loss appears, for instance, with Helen Keller's broken doll, the pig's sacrifice by the Polynesian tribe, as well as in Freud's story about Ernest, his grandson, who in playing "Fort! Da!" – "Gone! There!" – throws away the cotton reel and loses it for some seconds, in order to generate a lost – returned structure.

In Lévi-Strauss's own personal myth, too, object loss can be seen to inaugurate the subject. Lévi-Strauss held a myth in which, as a young boy, he had wanted to be a musician. But he was unable to follow through because he lacked a musical ear. So, it is no coincidence that in his later work with myths he used signifiers associated with music.

Subjectivity, Exchange, and Delayed Gratification

The first act of exchange consists of giving up the Real for the Symbolic. In other words, the first act of exchange occurs in the wake of a loss, and this loss forms the basis for the exchange of signifiers. To illustrate: the child gives up on being his mum's baby because a little brother has been born, but in return he now is "big brother". He renounces something actual ("mummy's baby" does in actual fact get a more thorough and exclusive treatment) and gains something symbolic (the title "big brother"). Later on, he will forego something symbolic for something else symbolic: from being the big brother, to becoming the husband of his wife. Primary repression occurs with the substitution of the signifier for the object itself. Secondary repression consists of the replacement of one signifier by another. Each such iteration refers back to the original act of substitution.

Exchange produces value that relies on delayed gratification – which in turn constitutes the core element of all cultural phenomena. We might say that the project we call "culture" rests on this deferral alone: desire instead of satisfaction. So crucial is the absence required for motion, that whenever it does not present itself naturally, it must be made to appear deliberately. It may take the shape of a cultural ceremony like Jewish circumcision, the "land-diving" or bungee practiced on Vanuatu, or the ritual breaking of a tile when people move into a new home, all these rites of passage include an act of cut, rupture, or loss. The ritualistic representation of the lack.

A similar function can be found in psychic symptoms, as illustrated here: A patient, currently in his second marriage, is trying to be a kind of father to his wife's children; she, too, tries to be a mother to his children, and together they are doing their best to be a complete family. Because the son of his wife was having a hard time, my patient cancelled a trip abroad. On digging a little deeper, it turns out that there was no real need for this, something of which he could have rendered himself account. He ignored the fact that his sacrifice could have been avoided, because he wanted it, following the logic: "A good father makes sacrifices for his children." Thus, cancelling the trip was an act of adoption. And how does the patient explain to himself that he was adopting his wife's son? By telling himself that he was making a sacrifice for his new role as a father. If this sacrifice of his were to be proven superfluous, it might "destroy the transaction," undoing, as it were, the exchange which would inaugurate him as father. This however is not the case. He is inaugurated as father by dint of his willingness to sacrifice, his intention – regardless of any actual need for it. It is through this sacrifice that the subject emerges, in this example the subject "father."

References

Freud, S. (1905). Three essays on the theory of sexuality. In J. Strachey (Ed. & Trans.) *The standard edition of the complete psychological works of Sigmund Freud* (Vol. 7, pp. 123–246). Hogarth Press.

Freud, S. (1920). Beyond the pleasure principle (J. Strachey, Trans.). In J. Strachey (Ed. and Trans.), *The standard edition of the complete psychological works of Sigmund Freud* (Vol. 18, pp. 1–66). Hogarth Press.

Keller, H. (1903). *The story of my life*. Doubleday, Page & Co.

Lacan, J. (1970–1971) *The seminar of Jacques Lacan XVIII: On a discourse that might not be a semblance* (C. Gallagher, Trans.). Unpublished manuscript.

Chapter 3

Meaning

Yehuda Israely

According to structuralism, things only gain meaning in a context. I mentioned how we can probe the meaning of the totem of a certain tribe only when we relate to myths about the totem animal's relations with other totem animals. Similarly, a word achieves meaning only in the context of the language in which it functions and then gains further meaning by being part of the individual's inner contextual fabric. Here is one way we may conceive of this: since signifiers have no existence outside context, language must have come into the world suddenly, at one blow.

In the previous chapter we saw how Helen Keller entered language, experiencing a hitherto unprecedented vitality flooding her world. Helen Keller's encounter with language, too, could not have taken off with one single word. This is why the presence of the doll as object and signifier was necessary. If the signifier "water" had appeared in isolation she would not have been able to understand it. To understand the principle of the link between word and object Helen needed at least two signifiers. The logical structure that renders meaningful the link name-thing looks as follows: the word "jug" stands to the feel of the grainy surface of ceramics as the word "water" to the sense of wet. At least two pairings between object and signifier are required to deduce the principle. Without encountering at least one more signifier – like "doll" or "jug" – Helen would have been unable to grasp the nature of the signifier. So, this structure of the sentence whose signifiers validate and give meaning to each other is shared by all cultural phenomena, whether it is spoken language, myth, kinship, or music, dance, and gastronomy.

Here I will illustrate how in the case of exogamous kinship relations, too, "exchange relations" had to emerge all at once. Exogamy, marriage between partners who do not belong to the same group, took off from the exchange of sisters between nuclear families. Only at a later stage was the taboo extended to all women from the same clan. Exogamy had to start from at least two marriages, a plurality of steps rather than a single one. Lévi-Strauss assumed that the exchange of sisters initially took place within the extended family, when one man gave away his sister to his cousin while the latter reciprocated by gifting his sister. The first exogamous wedding must therefore have

DOI: 10.4324/9781003773764-4

consisted of two parallel ceremonies, including four elements: two brothers and two sisters, with each brother getting married to the other's sister. It was a wedding conducted in the form of a transactional agreement.

The Quartet of Meaning – Analogy of Opposites

In his book, *The Elementary Structure of Kinship Relations* (1969) Lévi-Strauss wonders about the minimal unit of social relationships, i.e., where membership carries meaning, and which can be reproduced as such. Again, like in the case of water and jug, or of the two wedding ceremonies, this unit includes four elements. Exogamous exchange, like any other type of exchange, is performed on the basis of congruence that enables substitution: insertion in the same position in the structure. This type of congruence is caught by the word "like" or "as": "Just as my sister is for you, so is your sister for me." In the story of Helen Keller, we can observe structurally based exchange of this kind when the following words attain meaning: "Like the word 'water' stands for the sensation of wet, so the word 'jug' stands for the feel of touching the object that is a jug."

Though meaning emerges from four elements, this requires a prior process including various developmental stages. To learn to count up to four, as exchange requires, zero, one, two, and three must be acquired first. Below I discuss the typical form of each of these numbers as they appear in cultural studies: the "zero signifier" refers to the undefined thing; the signifier "one" – the "unary trait" supports circumscription, definition, and characterization; the "binary trait" produces concepts grounded in opposites, and finally, there is analogy, which, consisting of two opposites, generates meaning.

Mana and the Zero Signifier – Signifier Without Signified

The Trobriand Islands are situated between New Guinea and Australia, part of the so-called Kula ring. The exchange of gifts between the islanders follows a set of very clear rules: shell-disc necklaces are traded counter-clockwise when the traveler heads west, while shell bracelets are handed out clockwise, when they are eastbound (Malinowski 1922). The recipient of a gift holds on to it for a period that is neither too long nor too short, and then passes it on to someone else, on another island. Passing on the gift, the person recounts its story: what adventures and troubles they met on the way, the waves and the sharks they had to fight. Stories told by earlier givers, who gave the gift to the current individual, are also included. Thus, narratives covering generations of givers from the entire archipelago circulate. Each act of gifting enfolds chains of stories.

This tradition of Trobriand gift circulation was studied by Marcel Mauss, the earlier mentioned, extremely influential teacher of Lévi-Strauss (1961). Mauss understood that the gifts had no intrinsic value: they were used for the purpose of exchange alone. They served as a wave carrying the stories; they were, in effect, the goods being passed around. The object holds the story of the adventure of the giver, and of all of those who came before them. As such it serves as the basis for an ongoing conversation about adventures and comradeship. We might liken this to what interior designers call a "conversation piece": an object in the room whose role it is to spark a conversation. The object is there to create the true gift: conversation and connection between people.

The fact that the value of the gift seemed to inhere in the act of exchange as such led Mauss to probe the meaning of the Polynesian word *mana*, a word whose use was so widespread that it was hard to pinpoint its meaning. Some anthropologists before him had taken the word to stand for "magic," but Mauss thought this fell short of capturing the full range of its significance. *Mana*, he believed, was "something," in other words: anything. It denoted the undefined thing, called "something" without determining its nature, and the word was used to indicate "undefined."

The gift that circulates among the islands, like *mana*, can be anything. It can convey any story at all. *Mana* is a signifier that can carry any signified, an expression that performs the very bond between all members of the community.

This signifier-without-signified, Lévi-Strauss calls "zero-signifier" and it signifies agreement that signifiers have meaning, prior to us knowing the meaning of any specific signifier. The "zero commandment," not included in the Ten Commandments, stipulates: "You must listen to and follow." Lacan calls this function the Name of the Father. Freud's Oedipal myth describes the child's passage from the mother to the father. The Oedipal myth, for Lacan, offers a metaphor for the child's shift from a primitive state of being part of nature, into participation in the symbolic domain of language. The Name of the Father, therefore, represents both passage into the world of words and names, as well as the relationship of this passage to other, similar shifts: that from nature to culture, and from mother to father.

The father, who is the first substitute, gives his name to the principle of exchange and function as it's guarantee. The Name of the Father affirms: "Let's treat words as though they were things" and it functions to underwrite the meaning of words. When a language scholar comes across a stone with scratched markings, she will assume they bear meaning even if she doesn't know what that meaning is. This is the nature of digital coins too. Those who accredit them are in charge of their value. If they didn't the currency would be worthless – much like a story nobody cares to hear. The Trobrianders, hence, treat their shells as objects of exchange, much like we do with money.

The role of the zero-signifier is key to mental functioning. A baby will call everything "that!" before starting to sort the world into objects carrying definitions. The clinical implication of attending to the zero-signifier is that when it is part of the conversation there is, for now, no need to know the meaning of "that." We may tell the patient: "Just let 'that' be!," we may say: "Why not pick up on 'that'?," without having to know what "that" refers to. This is the subject of Lacan's (1954–1955) analysis of Edgar Allan Poe's "Purloined Letter" in which the queen is keeping a certain letter hidden from the king. The king sends his minister to steal the letter. Dupin, a private detective, steals the letter from the minister, returns it to the queen, and that's the end of the affair: we will never know the contents of the letter. The letter, then, is a type of "that": we need not know anything about its contents for the story to work. Like the shells passing hands among the islanders. "That" generates something due to its passing hands alone. We don't really need to know what it is that we are circulating: participating in the process of circulation itself is what matters.

The Unary Trait – One and Coincidence

If the zero-signifier announces, "It is valid!," then the signifier "one" or as it is also known, "the unary trait," states: "there is one!" Zero precedes one to make possible the statement: "one is valid!" How does "one" enter the world? And what does this conceptualization named "one" mean? A thing that stands out as such can be called "one." Something that has an outline and whose inside and outside differ. Here we have this one thing that is unlike everything else. This is, in other words, an act of isolation. In saying "one" we isolate something from everything else. It is a human act occurring nowhere else in nature. To isolate phenomena and call something a "unit" we need a signifier. You could think of the world as a thick broth, with humans using a ladle that allows us to scoop up one distinct ladleful which we define as separate from the remaining broth. The "unitary trait" is the ladle. It is the tool of the one-ness.

"Get us ten fruits. Any fruits. And in addition, five oranges and four apples" – this is an instruction given to a robot. Having arrived at the vegetable section in the supermarket the robot processes the data. It identifies objects in space, including fruits and vegetables. It puts a virtual sticker on every object and having scanned all the objects it proceeds to "write" the words "fruit," "orange," or "apple" on the labels. Oranges and apples, obviously, are also tagged as "fruits," while the labels on the vegetables stay empty. The robot collects ten pieces of fruit, five oranges, and four apples and continues shopping. The unary trait, in this illustration, is the sticker or label. It is what defines objects as countable.

What is the difference between the zero signifier and the unary trait? The zero signifier defines any object as such, as an object. The unary trait announces that the object is not just any object: it is specific, comes with a name, belongs in a category. What name and category, we don't know for now. It will be up to us to decide. We will determine, later on, whether this orange is one of the five oranges or one of the ten fruits. An "instance" is something we have isolated from the world as an "instance." It may be an instance of the "fruit" type, or of the "orange" one. The unary trait produces the singularity whereby one thing is singled out from its surroundings, it produces the "incidence."

The concept of "co-incidence" refers to how we apply the unary trait in defining things as either identical or different, as "the same" or not the same. Depending on how we define the instance or incidence, we join instances or incidents together into co-incidences. Here's a segment of a conversation to illustrate:

- Imagine what a coincidence! I'm zapping between TV stations and wherever I look, they're talking about the same subject: tables.
- Yes, I also experienced a coincidence. Whichever station I switched on – it was all about furniture: chairs, tables, wardrobes…
- Oh, but that's nonsense. If you saw tables and chairs that doesn't mean coincidence! A table and a chair – they're not the same thing.
- You decided that the incident was a table. And that one table and another table – that they're coincidence. But I decided that a piece of furniture is what constitutes an incidence, and so one piece of furniture and another make up a coincidence.

To begin with we determine the instance or incidence on the basis of what was added on, and then we announce the miracle of coincidence. "Coincidence" is a kind of rigged game.

"One" also captures how we refer to ourselves as a singularity, as a special instance or incidence, and how we perceive ourselves as distinct from our surroundings. In Lacanian developmental theory, one becomes part of the young child's self-perception in the mirror stage, as the child faces the mirror. The mirror image offers the child, who until that point experienced itself as a jumble of fragments, the possibility to identify with the reflection of its own outline, as body image and ego. The mirror image enables us to be an entity.

To be someone, to be something, we identify with "one." And we persuade ourselves that "one" is natural and a given premise, while in fact it is a signification, generated by language and cognition. Other animals don't seem to ascribe singularity to themselves in the way humans do when they use language. A mouse probably does not consider itself a mouselike entity (Lacan 1988) in any way comparable to human subjects.

"One" arose about a million and a half years ago with the emergence of the common shape of the hand-held ax. Until then, each ax looked different, either a little or much. Whoever chiseled himself a tool would follow his own hunch. The classical model of the tip did not exist, a stone rounded where the hand was to grip the tool and sharpened on the other side. But from a certain moment in pre-history, tools began to take a common, unified shape: this is what an ax looks like, this – a hammer, and this – a knife. Pre-historians assume it was the emergence of the mental ability to conserve a shape or model, which could then be repeated time after time, which was responsible for this change. Something in the human imagination matured to allow it to hold the form in mind, so that next time a person produced a tool they used this model. This model uses the unary trait to state: here's another one, that is to say: another one of the same thing; the consistency of the form making it qualify as "the same thing." "Another one" is also the incision the hunter made on his spear for each additional bison or antelope he caught – making the unary trait the origin of counting.

The Spatial Fiction of Identity and the Letter

Here I should admit that when introducing the unary trait, my definition was imprecise as I used a spatial metaphor distinguishing a form from a background – something that can be observed, for instance, when the child identifies itself as an entity standing out from the background it sees in the mirror. The unary trait, however, rather than being spatial, is symbolic. The child's identification with its reflection in the mirror is imaginary and it is developmentally crucial, but the unary trait is symbolic in nature, not imaginary. The image functions as an icon, a visual signifier, like a hieroglyph or a symbolic element that consists of images but could just as well have been made up out of sounds or objects. We may consider the peel of an orange which spatially sets it apart from its surroundings as what defines it as one, but we may also choose to count pairs of oranges, and here it is just our arbitrary choice that determines each pair as one countable entity. The operation that relates to people as spheres, i.e., separate and distinct from each other in the manner of oranges (with their peel forming a clear outline) is an imaginary effect but nonetheless of crucial importance. And if we already stick to spatial outlines, our digestive tract bestows on us the geometrical form of the doughnut-shaped torus. Because we identify with our mirror image, we define ourselves, however mistakenly, as spheres, but the unary trait defines us as distinct entities on the basis of a trait rather than in spatial terms. A pregnant woman, therefore, can be considered either one or two, depending on how we use language, and a person who misses a limb will not be thought of as less than one.

In contrast with the unified figure in the mirror, which sustains the illusory distinction between inside and outside, the words we use originate outside ourselves and return there when we speak. Some young children, and psychotic adults occasionally believe that their thoughts are being read. In so far as language belongs to all, they are right. It is not exclusively located either inside or outside the individual. The inside-outside distinction is irrelevant in regard to language. The store of signifiers and signs exists inside and outside simultaneously.

How Do We Read Myth?

Lévi-Strauss introduced the notion of the "binary trait," or "binary opposition" to describe his observation that cultures organize their world view and their social structures through pairs of opposites, with each such pair constituting a concept. The concept of "temperature," for instance, is generated by the pair of heat-cold, when playing at associations, and people are asked to respond rapidly with an opposite, many will come up with "cat" when asked to produce the opposite to "dog," or "table" when the cue is "chair." Here convention is more transparent. Lévi-Strauss argued that even where the binary's contents are conventional, humans' mode of perception, which divides the world into pairs, is not arbitrary and is a cultural universal.

An opposition which occurs in almost all myths, more or less cross-culturally, is the one between nature and culture, the movement from nature to culture and the articulation of cultural concepts through symbols from the natural world. Myths of creation directly engage this binary.

When we investigate a myth, we look at how it characterizes, isolates, and defines an idea by means of a comparison with (or likening to) pairs of opposing natural elements. This is how myth operates. It deploys nature-related symbols to say something about human beings. Here is an example: "moiety" or "half," is a form of exogamy practiced by some natives on the American continent, whereby the clan is subdivided into two halves, and marriage can only take place with a member of the other half of the clan. In the myth supporting the principle of moiety, the world was divided into two halves – sky and land, or sun and moon – and each half of the clan is mythically represented by one side of the natural opposition. In one myth, the sun and the moon once were brothers who became embroiled over a woman. They went their separate ways, and ever since one ruled over the realm of day, and the other over the night. By identifying one half of the clan with the sun, or alternatively with the moon, marriage between the earthly representatives of the sun and the moon imitates the cosmic reconciliation between the heavenly bodies. The mythic characters are like phonemes which only assume meaning as they come together into words. The sun, symbol of moiety, is meaningless outside the context of the myth about the relations between sun and moon, even as phonemes and letters remain meaningless without the context of other letters. Relationship is the primary entity of meaning. This is true for the family too: its key element are the relationships between people, not people as such. The minimal basic unit of myth, the minimal requirement for myth to exist, therefore, consists of four elements – two pairs and an analogy between them.

What holds for patterns of thinking in language, in the myths and kinship relations of primitive peoples, is also true for the speech patterns, dreams, and symptoms of human beings, even those who participate in modern culture. This is important in clinical work where symptoms function like a type of meaning-making myths, while they are, at the same time, a source of suffering. In therapy, the fourfold analogies that generate meaning present themselves constantly. One objective of psychoanalytic interpretation is to lay bare the unconscious meaning that is a structural element of the symptom, like

Lévi-Strauss did for the natives' myth. But our aim is not just to investigate the symptom; we want to dissolve it and remove its meaning, or at least replace it with an analogical quartet that, while supporting similar meaning, does not produce the suffering of the symptomatic analogy.

Here is a clinical illustration: a patient who has been promoted to a managerial position says the role of manager stands to that of their employee as victimizer to victim. Managerial work, therefore, is tantamount to tormenting or harassing one's employees. So, he does not wish to be a manager. The analogy, based on the victimizer/victim dyad, prevents him from taking on the job. If he could have said: manager stands to employee as father stands to son, he might have been able to deal with it. Why does the analogical function carry this particular meaning? We must find out. From whom did the patient inherit this meaning, this analogy? And what can we do to question it? We want to expose the analogy and free ourselves from it. We would like to think that things need not be this way.

And here is another clinical moment: a patient says, "My father doesn't take me seriously. He talks condescendingly about 'those military types' who brag about their ranking, and who get worked up about all that nonsense – but I am a senior officer." Later he tells me that "my father left the army with a sense of failure." The father's personal myth includes, in the manner of all myths, two basic pairs: there's the person who is successful – and works hard, and there's one who is a loser and a hedonist. The father identifies with the position of the hedonistic loser, foregrounding the latter. He says: What's the point of the effort? Better to be lazy, forget about all that work and enjoy yourself, even if in terms of success, it means failure. Success stands to effort, as failure to pleasure – the model is gain and cost. Success is gain, and effort is cost, and on the same lines pleasure is gain, and failure is cost. Therapy aims to reveal the father's desire to the son: your father would have to believe in this myth to come to terms with his own failure. He tells you: "Success is for those poor suckers who are trying so hard, while I am taking it easy, just enjoying myself, and that shows you it's worth the failure." Your father has had to believe that this pleasure is exclusively reserved for losers: it's his way of beating those hard-working achievers. But you're not obliged to live by this myth. It's not necessarily your choice. Couldn't you be a high achiever who is working hard and enjoying himself? Couldn't you take pleasure in the effort? Can you refuse your father's equation?

And here is a third example, this time in the form of a dream told by one of my patients: she finds herself stuck in a high spot from which she cannot move because down there, it's teeming with little snakes and worms. The association she has in the clinic is with earlier dreams when she experienced fear of heights. Interpretation begins with identification of the opposition and of the desire as formulated by the dream's scriptwriter. When interpreting dreams, we seek the desire – not that of the main actor, who is having to struggle with the dream's reality, but of the scriptwriter who invented that reality. What is this desire of the scriptwriter which the dream satisfies? What made the scriptwriter put up an obstacle that makes it impossible for the actor to come down? Since it is her dream we relate to her as the scriptwriter, as the subject of the unconscious, and ask her what made her do this. The wish is to stay up there, and the obstacle enables this, not because she chose to do so but because of "certain constraints." Since she complains about these constraints, she need not acknowledge the fact that this is about a wish. Rather than saying: "I want to be high up" she prefers to complain: "I have no choice but to stay up in this high spot." We note that she holds on to this high position while denying that it's her choice to be there. The dream presents the achieved desire, which is the desire to stay up high. "You create an obstacle for yourself, and it serves as a pretext for staying up high."

The split between the scriptwriter and the actor enables her to pursue what she wants, staying "up," without having to admit this wish. What then is this height the patient experiences as illicit and where she wants to stay, nevertheless? At this point we can identify three out of four elements that make up the pairs in the analogy. She was asked: high stands to low, like X stands to little snakes. She replied: "To do great things." The following statement renders the complete quartet: "High stands to low much like a person who does great things stands to small animals." In other words, the meaning of what she calls "being stuck up there" is the thing she feels uncomfortable acknowledging, namely, doing big things as opposed to what the little snakes do. These little snakes fulfil a two-fold role. They constitute the opposite to "big things," while at the same time also presenting the obstacle by means of which she can choose to occupy this high spot, pretending she's afraid while this is her choice. Making this choice explicit would clash with her taboo against superiority

Additional opposites suggest themselves if we want to continue the interpretation. Do the worms contribute anything over and beyond the snakes? Are they just some more small things? Or do they carry a singular meaning, to contrast with certain human attributes? For instance: "Unlike these disgusting worms, I am an attractive woman, and unlike the maggots who can be associated with a dead corpse, I am alive!" We will only know whether these hypothetical possibilities are relevant if we continue listening to the patient's associations. Neither snakes nor worms, it must be stressed, have inherent meaning – just as letters in a word don't mean anything in isolation. Meaning is contextual, so that we must relate to the dream as if it were structured like a myth involving snakes and worms, if we wish to say something about it. The psychoanalyst must be attentive to the context of the signifiers and images, or else they will be imposing their own private content disguised as symbols with absolute meanings, in an act of interpretation grounded in predetermined archetypes.

Between Diachronic Narrative and Synchronic Structure

The narrative aspect of a myth is inherently diachronic, unfolding along a timeline, as it involves the sequence of events and actions that develop over time. In contrast, the synchronic dimension pertains to the structural aspects of the myth, which exist beyond the timeline. The synchronic structure represents the underlying relationships, patterns, and systems that organize the myth, offering a timeless framework within which the diachronic narrative operates. If we approach dreams like myths, we should keep in mind that myths have different versions, and that a myth's meaning also flows from the relations between these versions.

If we conclude that the worms, in the above dream, are not just another small creature, like the snakes, but carry additional meaning, we will say it presents a different version of the same myth, and we will try to figure out what meaning this version contributes to the dream.

Let's zoom in on the relations between the diachronous and synchronous story: there is the narrative of a particular story, and there is the story of how the versions evolved. For instance, say you went to see a film; you understand its story with its particular plot. Then another director decides to create another version of the story, which takes a different angle. The diachronic aspect is the narrative of the one specific version, while the synchronic aspect refers to the plurality of versions in existence at any point in time. Each version adds or changes something. If snakes and worms are one and the same thing, we end up with only one version. But if the worms add something to the story, which would have remained outside of it had the story's meaning only included the snakes, then here we have another version. If the patient associates "worms" with "maggots, death," then the earlier opposite – big human vs small animal – expands to big, living human vs small, and associated with death. This represents yet another change in the story. There is no final, complete synchronous story. Any attempt to tell the ultimate story stops at "just one more version" – casting further light on one more aspect. Still – if we were not driven to "say everything," we might lose the motivation to say anything at all.

Lévi-Strauss offered a geometric representation of the narrative of one myth vs other versions of that myth along Cartesian coordinates – a horizontal and a vertical axis. The x-coordinate is the diachronic one representing the story of the myth. It is horizontal in the same sense as it is written: a sentence consisting of words linked to each other, with each added word changing the meaning, including that of the words preceding it. The y-coordinate can be likened to a skewer that pierces right through a pile of stacked papers: each sheet holds another version of the myth.

The Cinderella myth, for instance, has many versions, featuring diverse small animals. In the Grimm brothers' version, they are birds that help Cinderella finish her chores so she will be in time for the ball. In the French version, these are mice; in the Italian, lizards; the Scots have dogs, the Chinese, fish, while Walt Disney's U.S. version turns them into mice. The skewer is the motif, or mytheme: the myth's basic unit. So, the mytheme "small animals" passes, like a three-dimensional vector, through the two-dimensional sheets of paper, through the different versions told by various communities, featuring different types of "small animals." If we want to understand the differences between the versions, we need to know the cultural connotation of the specific small animal in any group's version. In the Chinese version, the small animals are fish, and they symbolize good fortune, while for the French, mice connote resourcefulness. The choice of different animals expresses the particular cultural values and variations of the narrative on the structure of the myth.

References

Lacan, J. (1954–1955). Seminar on 'The Purloined Letter' (B. Fink, Trans.). In J. Lacan, *Écrits: The First Complete Edition in English* (pp. 6–48). W. W. Norton & Company.

Lacan, J. (1988). *The seminar of Jacques Lacan, Book IX: Identification* (D. Porter, Trans.). W. W. Norton & Company.

Lévi-Strauss, C. (1969). *The elementary structures of kinship* (J. H. Bell, J. R. von Sturmer, & R. Needham, Trans.). Beacon Press.

Malinowski, B. (1922). *Argonauts of the Western Pacific: An account of native enterprise and adventure in the archipelagoes of Melanesian New Guinea*. Routledge & Kegan Paul.

Chapter 4

Kinship Relations

Yehuda Israely

There's a joke about a three-year-old boy who has never uttered a word, and now suddenly turns to his mother: "Can you please pass the salt?" When his mother asks him how come he has suddenly started speaking, and what stopped him from doing so before, he replies: "The salt was never missing till now." Here we can see language serving in lieu of the actual thing. Lacan said about this that the word killed the thing. With regard to myth, similarly, the group's shared story replaces unprocessed experience.

Kinship relations were another domain Lévi-Strauss investigated by means of his structural method. While in the domain of language, the basic, meaningful unit is the word, and in myth, the mytheme, then in kinship relations the human individual is "the thing." We may say that as "the word kills the thing," in kinship relations roles substitute for individuals. But here, maybe because the human individual itself is at issue, it is harder to identify the language-like nature of these phenomena. Still, we will nevertheless turn our attention to how the principle of joining arbitrary elements to yield a meaningful sign evolves in the case of kinship relations, and how Lacan's statement about the substitution of the word for the thing applies here too.

The elementary unit that serves to attribute social roles to people is exogamy (i.e., marrying out: outside the family, the clan, the tribe), which in its most rudimentary form consists of two men marrying each other's sister. In this form of exogamy, each man takes the role of both husband, brother, and brother-in-law, and the same holds for the two women. Just like a letter out of the context of a word has no meaning, a person outside a kinship structure has no meaning – for others.

In kinship relations, more than in other language- or culture-based practices, renunciation of the object in the transition to language is particularly marked. The pleasure of incestuous relations is undeniably curbed for the sake of social ties. People's social roles hold their incestuous-autoerotic impulses in check, impulses driving entropically towards the social structure's dissolution.

DOI: 10.4324/9781003773764-5

Entropy and Anti-Entropy – The Principle of Delayed Gratification

Entropy refers to the degree of disorder in a system. The law of entropy holds that systems constantly approach a state of disorder; while preserving structure, its complexity and order require a steady investment of energy. Atoms join into simple molecules, which link up with complex DNA molecules, which in turn come together and form cells. Cells compose multi-cellular creatures, which then assemble into ecological communities and systems. The system's level of complexity rises with each consecutive stage. Passing from a lower to a higher level of complexity requires energy. When, by contrast, a system falls apart into a lesser degree of complexity, energy is released. This metaphor from the domain of physics also works for processes of social organization. A rise in the level of social organization requires that the individual invest energy in delaying gratification. When an inverse process, of reduced complexity, takes place – as when agreements are canceled or norms are broken, lowering the level of social organization – the resulting release of energy will be felt as a discharge of pleasure. In return for the individual's willingness to delay the gratification, society offers another type of gratification: that of community ties and the benefits associated with complex exchange processes. To put it more specifically: as the individual enters kinship relations – the subject of the present chapter – they must give up autoerotic pleasure to be received into the familial structure, and this entails a variety of gains.

Freud's pleasure principle (1920) is about the entropic quest of the inanimate to return to its basic state. To dismantle the biological level of organization and revert to an inanimate state. Freud's metaphor, we might observe, took the Biblical "from dust thou camest and to dust thou shalt return" and transformed it into: "dust seeks to revert to dust," thereby adding his own version to the familiar myth in an attempt to illustrate the phenomenon of entropy in the psychic dimension. Human regression, according to Freud, does not stop at the wish to return to infancy. The yearning for nirvana – the equivalent to the human death wish – is nothing but the inorganic wanting to be restored to itself. It is as if the death drive Freud described in "Beyond the Pleasure Principle" is how the inorganic asserts itself within the human.

Contemporary physicist Jeremy England (2014) has been called the "new Darwin" because he discovered the "anti-entropic" dynamics typical of living creatures are also present in inanimate atoms. The living creature invests energy, which it harvests from its surroundings to prevent the disintegration of its molecules, and the release or loss of energy stored in the links between atoms. Even inanimate entities, England found, operate according to the principle of delayed gratification, when, under certain conditions, they try to conserve energy. Sometimes molecules organize themselves to maximize absorption and release of energy in the form of heat, though in the short term this form of organization would require an investment of energy. This discovery blurs the distinction between animate and inanimate or at least describes the appearance of initial living molecules from an anti-entropic feature already existent in inorganic matter. What would Freud have said if England had told him he had chosen the wrong metaphor for the human drive toward nirvana.

What England discovered about anti-entropic processes on the inorganic level can show us that exogamy is part of a more extensive phenomenon. The human community's level of organization turns out to be just another expression of the law of nature aiming for energy efficiency. This is a metaphysical approach which grounds the law of human energy efficiency, forming the basis of exogamy, as well as the advantages of highly evolved exchange relations, in a natural law, which obtains in the physical world as well as in the passage from physical to biological. Molecules, like humans, will tend to reduce present energy output for rationalization purposes by joining into larger systems.

Creation myths deal with this anti-entropic leap from nature to culture, from the auto-erotic to exchange relations, and from the struggle for ownership of the female family members to the organized exchange of brides that is exogamy. Exogamy, aiming for marriage outside the family, and eventually the tribe, institutes a higher level of social organization and the result is that the community, serving as the framework for exchange relations, grows larger and more sophisticated.

Anguish and Moving Between Levels of Organization

One explanation of anxiety is that it appears at junctions of dimensional leaps between levels of organization. At such moments, castration anxiety appears. Castration represents the foregoing of gratification, the price a person pays for this change in dimension. Another way of putting this is that one must forgo gratification for the sake of desire. While pleasure takes the form of gratification of direct individual needs, desire is the outcome of the individual's mission or function in the broader system. Joining this system always involves giving up private pleasure. Where we encounter anxiety, we must look for the next level of organization the person is facing, whether the context is that of the family or any other organization. What is the next dimension that the subject is hesitant to enter? What is the price in terms of personal pleasure, and what is the gain in the domain of desire for a protagonist living their narrative in their community?

When one must reluctantly forgo a pleasure when entering social exchange this expresses itself in distress or anguish. James Strachey translated the German *Angst* as *anxiety*, but Lacan preferred the word *anguish*: anguish is "the lack of the lack," meaning that a place meant to be empty has become blocked. Something has become excessive or superfluous. The anguish experienced at a shift in dimension is due to the difficulty in letting go of an object at a lower level of organization. This difficulty on the cusp of change causes the object to become a source of anguish. In the transition, for instance, from the position of the baby immersed in the gratification of her or his needs, to the position of the child who enters exchange relations, the child has to give up their direct relation with their mother, while it now earns the title "big one." The bond with the mother is symbolized by the breast. The object "breast," which must be relinquished for the sake of turning into a "big one" transforms over time into an anguishing object. Witness the four-year old's embarrassment about still using a pacifier. The word "anguish" conveys the effect of excess where there should be lack. What used to be satisfying becomes overwhelming.

In "Mourning and Melancholia" (Freud 1957), Freud explains that depression is unresolved mourning. Depression and anguish share a refusal to let go of the object. The depressed person, however, follows the lost object into the grave, just like Hamlet did with Ophelia, while the anxious person continues to carry the object who gives him anguish, like a mourner who carries the body of his deceased lover wherever he goes.

The Political Expression of the Conflict in Levels of Organization – Right Versus Left

The fundamental tensions constituting exogamy, much like the conflict sparked by the passage to a higher level of organization, occur on a higher dimension of organization, sociological and political, in the relations between groups and states, where they take the form of the tension between competition and collaboration, as these notions are defined in games theory. Will people lock themselves in an all-out war over resources or do they proceed to a higher level of social organization by maximizing general gains through cooperation? The answer to this question has far-reaching implications in many domains, starting with animal evolution down to political theory. How did wolves come to be domesticated into dogs? The assumption is that given their less evolved adrenal gland, wolves were less susceptible to fear and less aggressive when approaching human habitation, than their more sensitive siblings. This in fact explains not only how wolves became domesticated, but the process of domestication of all animals whose hormonal economy led to less fear and aggression, making them more amenable to forms of cooperation with humans. In the perception of dogs, humans came to feature as leaders of the group. From the human perspective, the relationship has quite a few overlaps with master–slave relations, but in evolutionary terms it's a symbiosis between partners. Domestication carries mutual benefits: dogs give humans protection against predators, and they receive leftover food from humans. During the hunt, dogs spot the prey, and humans shoot the arrow.

Since exchange and cooperation form the basis of liberal thinking, we may say that global culture is an improved and expanded form of the principle of exogamy. The liberal is more "domesticated" than the fundamentalist. Fundamentalist thought believes in power and considers the global world as apes' ongoing competition for alpha-male position. The founding element of liberal thought, by contrast, is the shared totem with its commonly agreed values. While fundamentalism allows strife and pulls towards war, liberalism aims for cooperation and freedom. Of course, these matters are more complex. Conflict is structural in western liberal culture, and capitalism can be seen as a contemporary version of tribal war, with corporations replacing tribes. Here the principle is that individual competition now dominates social relations, with the strong growing rich at the expense of the weak.

What then should we prefer? Right or left? Democrats or Republicans? We may find one answer in the domain of games theory. The more open we are to acts of exchange, to a more complex economy marked by less fear and more trust, less competition and more cooperation, gains will grow exponentially for all. But this will only work if everybody plays the game. As long as there are people who exploit others' trust with the aim of dominating and growing wealthy, they undermine the operation of exchange. Rather than human solidarity, what remains is *homo homini lupus est*.

Freud and Lévi-Strauss – On Incest and the Importance of Exogamy

Lévi-Strauss cites from Margaret Mead's research on the Arakesh tribe in Papua New Guinea. She recounts how her informer asked the native, "Why don't you marry your sister?," and he replied: "What's wrong with you? To marry your sister!? Don't you want to have a brother-in-law to go hunting with? Don't you realize that if you marry a man's sister and your sister marries another man, you have two brothers in law to hunt with, not to mention that they may have more brothers. If you marry your sister, you will not have even one" (Lévi-Strauss 1969 p. 485)

Lévi-Strauss understood this to reflect that the native believed the taboo's point was to spur exchange, which in turn came to encourage alliances and relationships between tribes and clans. This was what aristocratic families would do when they arranged marriages between princes and princesses from different countries to create or confirm alliances. In the same way as the Trobrianders exchanged shell-disc necklaces, the exchange of wives in marriage supports tribal relations. But the taboo served more than this one purpose: maintaining it was a matter of life and death. The natural thing, as it were, would be to grab hold of food, not share it and not risk getting involved in exchange. Edward Burnett Tylor, an anthropologist cited by both Freud and Lévi-Strauss, had already commented on this as early as 1871: "Marry out or be killed out" (Lévi-Strauss 1969 p. 43).

Giving up on their own clan's women, men gain access to all other unmarried women in the tribe, and beyond it. If men had not foregone their daughters and sisters and allowed them to be married off outside the family, they would have had to constantly protect and fight against any other men's unbridled claim on them. Traces of ritualized resistance to exogamy can still be observed in the ritual abduction of Caucasian brides.

Among apes, the war against the alpha male is not total. Chimpanzees engage in rituals of competition but usually do not actually kill each other in their attempt to claim a female. As soon as it is apparent who is the strongest, the fight ends in surrender. The human point of departure seems worse: in the absence of a structural arrangement like exogamy, ensuring non-competition, the struggle can escalate, much like it does between cannibalistic sharks, who will devour each other even in the womb. Something like this occurred among the Ottoman aristocracy where becoming the king's heir required killing one's siblings. The last surviving brother is crowned as the next king.

In effect, the taboo underlying the prohibition on sex within the family prohibits pleasure in a broader sense: delayed gratification enables us to protect each other from starvation. It evolved in parallel with the development of human intelligence, supporting the insight into how useful it is to delay; the same goes for exchange relations. Games theory shows us how exchange relations came to gain meaning: clans' move to the exchange of women promoted peaceful relations in a way not unsimilar to the introduction of the idea of nuclear detente. In the absence of trust, the stronger will exploit the weaker for the sake of small gains, but the gains increase tremendously where there is trust among all. When everyone trusts everyone, common gains increase. Foregoing ownership of your sister parallels giving up on doomsday arms for the sake of global peace.

Freud and Lévi-Strauss agreed that taboo was a human psychological and cultural phenomenon. They agreed that prohibition is crucial for the survival and continuation of family and tribe. They also agreed that the precedence of culture over nature, of collective over individual is what allows society to become organized into a structure that can be reproduced. Oedipal taboo allows a child to identify with their parent and reproduce the family, while the taboo on sibling marriage ensures the clan's continued existence by avoiding all-out war between alpha males. Where Freud and Lévi-Strauss differed is in the fact that while Freud believed that the prohibition on incest evolved from the prohibition against intercourse between parents and children, Lévi-Strauss focused on the prohibition against incest between siblings through exogamy, which regulates the relations between closest family and tribe, making possible a broader social structure.

Lévi-Strauss applied the principle of analogy to nearly every symbolic domain. As a reminder, language entered the world at one, distinct moment in time, and the minimal requirement for the emergence of meaning is the analogical quaternary. Now that we have gained a deeper understanding of the concept of exogamy, we may notice that it operates along, and supports, the same analogical structure: no one will give away his sister without receiving another woman in exchange: marriage between families or tribes, therefore, can never be one-sided – it is, by definition, reciprocal. Alliances must be mutual; this is an a priori agreement without which the act cannot be performed. The same can be said about words and signifiers in a language; they function because they mutually validate each other.

The Prohibition on Incest – Cultural or Genetic?

The native population of the Andaman Islands arrived 60,000 years ago when the archipelago was still connected to the Asian continent. They were among the first waves of homo sapiens leaving Africa. In some important ways, it is the currently most ancient, simple, and isolated culture. It is from this culture that Lévi-Strauss quoted a myth about incest.

This Andamanese myth has it that the future world, the utopian world of the spirits of the dead, will be like the present world in all respects except for two: everyone will stay young and healthy, at the peak of well-being, and there will be neither death nor decline; and there will be neither marriage nor the giving away of women in marriage (Lévi-Strauss 1969). Freedom from exogamy, in other words, is presented as the ultimate pleasure. The myth reflects awareness that the utopian phantasm of fullness, of unlimited pleasure, is essentially incestuous. Unlike their neurotic western counterparts, Andamanese natives feel no embarrassment about having such fantasies. They accept the taboo, reluctantly – culture comes at a price – but the desire is not yet repressed. Where there is no repression, and no failed repression taking the form of a symptom, there's no reason for neurosis. In psychoanalysis, too, which situates the taboo in the Oedipus complex, it is well known that incestuous fantasies feature as a pleasure reluctantly forgone.

Both Freud and Lévi-Strauss highlighted the structural effect of the prohibition of incest and tended to make little (if anything) of the role of natural/biological mechanisms aiming to protect the species against the transmission of genetic mutations caused by marriage between blood relations. Such mechanisms can be seen at work in nature – many male mammals tend to leave the pack on attaining sexual maturity and go in search of females in other packs. Domesticated animals, like cats, whose movement is limited, show more incestuous behaviors.

There is a diversity of cultural expressions of the taboo. The central African Azande tribe have the following saying: "The desire for the wife begins with the sister" (Lévi-Strauss 1969 p. 17). The prohibition on incest, in other words, is not instinctive, as far as they are concerned. We occasionally find traces of a time when sexual relations between brothers and sisters were not forbidden. In the royal pharaonic families of Egypt, and among the Polynesian royalty of Hawaii, marriages between siblings were not uncommon

(Ager 2021; Kirch 2019). But the fact that these incestuous practices were only allowed by exception, among the aristocracy can also be taken to suggest that incest was generally forbidden.

Though Freud foregrounded the taboo on incest as the cause of neurosis, there exist other, no less severe, taboos such as those on zoophilia and on necrophilia – phenomena that are human but rarely occur elsewhere in nature. In contrast, the incestuous act is not outside animal sexuality as is necrophilia. Only the human superego will not let it pass. The taboo on incest is the most conspicuous of a whole series of features marking the transition from nature to culture, all qualifying as "delayed gratification." Other instances are replacing the wish to be the only child by the pleasure of having siblings; reining in aggressive sibling rivalry; oral weaning, and anal control. Lacan, too, considers the Oedipally driven transition from mother to father as the key metaphor underlying the shift from nature to culture, and this is a principle with many manifestations over and beyond the Oedipus complex and the prohibition on incest.

Creation myths almost always start off with an incestuous scene – either directly or by using another metaphor describing a process of getting locked into a closed cycle. The myth's plot includes an act of resignation – abandoning a first stage and the irreversible move into a second one. In the first act of exchange, incestuous pleasure is given up, and in return for it, there is cultural creation.

The Myth of the Origin or Roasted Meat – The Price of Failed Exogamy and the Passage from Animal to Human

Two brothers-in-law belonging to the indigenous Bororo people in Brazil went into the forest to hunt for some parrot chicks whose feathers they were planning to use for the wedding outfit of the eldest of the two who was getting married to the younger one's sister. The younger brother-in-law climbed the ladder but didn't get hold of the chicks. Instead, he grabbed hold of two eggs and when he threw them down so the older one would catch them, they fell to the ground and transformed into two stones. Now they were useless, and this stopped the exogamous exchange relations. The older brother-in-law took the ladder and left. The younger one stayed stuck in the tree, and for lack of other food was forced to eat his own excrement.

The law of exogamy forms the background against which we must understand this myth about the brothers-in-law. Brothers-in-law were, originally, two men who exchange sisters through marriage. Initially exogamy aimed to achieve cooperation between the brothers-in-law. Only later on did exchange relations expand beyond the family and came to include tribes.

In the above myth the younger brother-in-law, who fails, is the one giving his sister at this particular wedding. He does not come up with the feathers necessary for the wedding. He does not keep his side of the agreement when he casts down the eggs that transform into stones. This metamorphosis might signify a denial of the meaning of fertility, which is substituted by violence. The elder man reacts by breaking his part of the agreement and removing the ladder. The vicious, auto-erotic cycle is symbolized by the younger man staying behind in the tree and having to eat his own feces. This is a metaphor for remaining within the incestual structure. "Incest" does not only mean having actual sexual intercourse with one's parent. Wherever a person is locked in a closed cycle with her or himself the situation is similarly regressive.

But let's go back and look further into the version of the myth I mentioned first (Lévi-Strauss 1990 p. 66): the younger man is still stuck in the tree, when a jaguar approaches. He returns the ladder, asks the man to climb down the tree and come home with him. The jaguar adopts the young man as his son, to the chagrin of his wife, who is half-jaguar, half-human. Picking up on the earlier regressive motifs, adoption into the jaguar's family represents regression from human culture into the animal domain. Next, the jaguar teaches the young man to use bow and arrows, an act symbolizing a first step towards cultural development as a result of forgoing regressive pleasure. The jaguar allows the young man to kill his wife – who in this narrative symbolizes the link between humans and animals. But why would the young man actually want to kill the jaguar's wife?

For an answer to this question, we must look to another myth from the Bororo (Lévi-Strauss 1990 p. 82). This myth tells the story of a girl who was fascinated by the jaguar's way of hunting for meat and wished to marry him. The girl became the jaguar's wife and developed jaguar-like traits: claws, fangs and so on. She was now part jaguar, part human. These myths tie into each other: the murder of the jaguar-woman by the young man is her punishment for having regressively preferred an animal over a human bridegroom. The young man's killing of the woman renders a logical negation of the link between animal and man – thus shifting the balance in favor of the transition to culture.

Later in the same myth in which the younger brother-in-law is rescued by the jaguar and taken home by him, the young man takes the meat the jaguar and his wife have cooked and shares it with his tribe. The tribe entered the jaguar's cave and took away the remaining meat as well as the fire. This is how the young man made up for his transgression against his exogamous partner, the older brother-in-law. The myth recounts how, ever since, humans have been roasting meat, while jaguars hate humans and eat raw meat.

Like many other myths of creation, this one aims to describe the creation of a cultural phenomenon: the cooking or roasting of meat. The price is the loss of humans' bond with animals, but the gain is that they now are cultural creatures.

Readers of myth should not be overly sensitive to murder. Death, in mythology, cancels, like negation in logic. The killing of the jaguar-woman removes doubt about the dividing line between animal and human, spelling the completion of the passage from animal to a human or cultural being. The jaguar woman represents an intermediate stage, between living being and speaking being, a link that will vanish to make space for the human and its maturation in culture. This has a parallel in the family myth where the nipple joins mother and child. Weaning from breast feeding and separation from the nipple constitute a stage in the process of the child's maturation. The pacifier, a version of the nipple, becomes a cast-off object, helping to reject the domain shared by mother and child, for the sake of transitioning from baby to child.

Avunculate – Father or Uncle? Stages Toward Full Exogamy

Exogamy really is a whole continuum in the sense that we can distinguish between cultures in terms of the degree and manner in which a sister passes from her brother to her husband's family. The relations between a woman and her husband are the inverse of those between a mother and her brothers: the closer a woman is to her husband, the more detached she will be from her brother, and the other way around: the closer she is to her brother, the more remote from her husband. She will never be equally close to both men – or equally detached from them. Culture prescribes that child always follows the mother, so that if a mother is closer to her brother, the child too will tend toward its uncle rather than father. Closeness will be reflected in a joking relationship, while detachment produces respect and fear.

Edvard Westermarck, a Finnish anthropologist, coined the term *avunculate* (referring to the Latin for maternal uncle) to denote the widespread cultural practice whereby an uncle – the mother's brother – serves as a father figure for her child, in most cases her sons as well as daughters. In Circassian society an uncle, rather than the father, may indeed act as the child's father figure: he is responsible for the child's education and has the authority to make decisions about its future. The avunculate can be considered a phase on the way to full exogamy. Even though the brother gave away his sister in an act of exchange, he still raises her son, so the sister has not entirely left her original family.

Prior to Lévi-Strauss's structural anthropology, there was functional anthropology, which interprets phenomena in terms of functions. For them, the uncle is the formal patriarch because the group does not trust the one who claims to be the child's father to necessarily be its biological father. In the case of the uncle, who is, after all, the mother's brother, at least on the mother's side. Genetic proximity is not in doubt. Lévi-Strauss, however, believed that the uncle does not simply serve to "patch up" this uncertainty: his status as formal patriarch is grounded in something more primitive. The uncle was there from the beginning, before the husband. It is he who instituted the family unit by exchanging sisters with another man. Among the Yoruba people in Nigeria, a hybrid form between the earlier mentioned Polynesian regressiveness, in the form of exempting the aristocracy from the prohibition on incest, and the avunculate, can be observed. Only among the nobility does the uncle function as a father figure in passing on the role of the chief: the son of the previous chief's daughter is his heir (Bascom 1969). Rather than the issue of trust between woman and man, exogamy addresses exchange in the group. When the uncle gives away his sister, yet not the sister's son, he thereby signals where the boundary of trust in exchange actually runs.

Exogamy and the Case of Dora

In the previous chapter, which was dedicated to the conditions necessary for the creation of meaning, we discussed the analogical structure in language: a stands to b, as c stands to d. In the language of kinship relations, the same structure produces exogamy: I stand to your sister as you to mine. We can read the case of Dora, one of Freud's earlier and most famous clinical cases, with reference to this same structure: Dora is part of a square-structured family including her father and the K.'s, a married couple. Lacan called this foursome Dora's "minuette." This quaternary structure played a critical role for Dora, in the sense of pouring meaning into her role as a woman (Freud 1905).

While Dora's father was having an affair with Mrs. K., Mr. K. tried to kiss 14-year-old Dora. When she asked him, "how dare you," Mr. K. replied: "But why not? You know that my wife means nothing to me." Dora slapped him in response. In the legal sense, what we have here is a case of sexual harassment of a minor, but Dora's reaction does not relate to that: it is about the way in which Mr. K. dissed his wife. Lacan refers to Dora's slap in his critique of Freud's view of the psychology behind her actions, as well as to introduce Lévi-Strauss' teachings about exogamy. Lacan interprets the case in terms of Dora's attempt to identify as a woman and sees the slap as the breakdown of that effort.

Dora was Freud's pseudonym for Ida Bauer, whose father brought her in for treatment in 1900, when she was 14 years old. He had found a suicide note among her things. She suffered from a variety of bodily complaints that Freud associated with repressed Oedipal conflict. He attributed her breakdown to her repressed feelings for Mr. K. These feelings of love, Freud thought, should be seen as her transferring her love for her father. Dora, however, repeatedly rejected this interpretation.

Deeming Freud's interpretation wrong, Lacan believed that his mistake was the result of countertransference. Lacan felt that Freud had misjudged his own blind spots in Dora's treatment. Identifying with the male positions in Dora's narrative, he included himself as another of her sexual objects. Her protests were of no avail; Freud could not budge from this perspective. Lacan approaches the case differently; he focuses on the moment when Dora's attitude to her father's affair changes. At some point Dora stops colluding with the affair and begins to oppose and even thwart it. For Lacan, this turn of events and Dora's slap are connected. Freud can be said to conceive this scene as part of a contemporary romantic comedy: first the girl slaps the guy, and then they kiss. The act only conventionally marks her refusal, because a nice girl is not supposed to go along too eagerly – no matter how much she wants the embrace. But Lacan looks at the way Dora went along with things until the moment of the slap in a very different light. He agrees with Freud who believed Dora was enabling her father's affair with Mrs. K. by getting close to her husband. But unlike Freud, Lacan thought that rather than reflecting on her attraction to Mr. K., it was about her identification with Mrs. K. Instead of Mr. K. himself, her object of interest is his desire. In Dora's structure, it is the man's desire, embodied in his gaze on the woman that designates her as such. Lacan argues that Dora realized something when Mr. K. told her his wife meant nothing to him. This statement caused the quaternary structure to fall apart, i.e., the analogical structure including the two men and the two women, which attributes certain roles to each of them.

This structure holds due to the role each member plays in relation to the others. When sisters are exchanged in the tribal context, each sister has a clear meaning or value for her brother, which is why giving her away in marriage is an act of surrender. The act is worthwhile since the man gets to marry the sister of another man and gains an ally in his new brother-in-law. The quaternary logic in Dora's story is identical: the family ties between the brothers are replaced by those between father and daughter, and between husband and wife. Here too, exchange is possible on the basis of the women's "value." Dora has produced a sense of identity from her place in the structure and reacts violently when the structure comes apart and her identity along with it.

Why did Dora need this quaternary structure to forge her female identity? Dora's mother was a weak and scorned figure. Taking no interest in her, her husband preferred having affairs with other women. The fact that he chose Dora's company over hers and decided to take her, instead of his wife, along on a vacation seemed incestuously tinged. Though this position of being her father's favorite female person seemed a sort of triumph in the Oedipal competition, it represented, simultaneously, a defeat, robbing Dora of the identification with the mother, she needed to establish herself as a valuable female person. She was an attractive girl, but this was no guarantee against her growing up into a rejected woman like her mother. Mr. K.'s advances, therefore, were not enough to ensure Dora's female identity (Voruz 2007). Dora's hysterical symptoms are related to an absence in the feminine signifier, something she is trying to acquire by observing Mrs. K. and trying to figure out, via Mr. K.'s gaze, what is feminine about her. What does he like about her, as a woman?

Going back to our earlier formula, Dora's meaning as a woman emerges through the analogy between opposites: a stands to b, as c stands to d. In Dora's unconscious the quaternary structure appears as follows: Mr. K. identifies me as a woman just like my father identifies Mrs. K. as a woman. But for this formula to work, there must be a parallel between the two men as well as between the two women. Exogamy works because sister and wife are parallels, hence subject to exchange. For Dora's father, Dora and Mrs. K., being both attractive women, can be exchanged. But it is not enough for Dora that her father identifies Mrs. K. as desirable. That would only suffice to justify the quaternary's existence. It is not from her father's gaze at Mrs. K. that Dora derives her sense of femininity, it is the structure that produces this effect. And when Mr. K. comments that Mrs. K. isn't worth anything, he destroys the structure. As her mother means nothing to her father, she sought for a woman whose femininity men identify as valuable as an object of identification. Once Mr. K. said: "she means nothing to me," he removed the reason for her efforts: "You cannot be an attractive woman to men, because Mrs. K. isn't an attractive woman to me." At the same time, he is also telling her: "I cannot supply you with a female figure of identification, because I don't attach value to her."

In Lacan's terms, Dora's slap is a "passage to the act," an eruption of the Real, as happens in the case of trauma. The fact that Dora's hand suddenly, intuitively went for Mr. K.'s face, without much thought, was as if to say: "When the symbolic structure collapses, the Real irrupts." If this had been Dora's communicative attitude we might have said that the slap was acting out some message, which could be put into words. But this is a moment without message, it is the collapse of messages.

Putting together Dora's story with Lévi-Strauss's myths, we remember the idea that for culture to develop, incestuous pleasure must be surrendered. Dora wants to do this, she is willing to lose the Oedipal struggle, let go of the regressive death drive of the oedipal victory and win in the battle for life, belonging to language and culture – losing out to a worthy rival, one with whom she can identify. She wants to be inferior to an admired mother – a role momentarily occupied by Mrs. K. – to have a chance, at some later point in time, to be a desirable woman herself. What a child really wants, and what the Amazonian native really wants, is to be human, namely, to forgo the pleasure of incest, and overcome the indistinction between themselves and nature. The jaguar woman, part human and part animal, must die in the passage to a meat cooking culture. Her death represents the logical negation of the intermediate stage, and the definitive break between nature and culture. What the human being eventually wants is for the connection with the mother to be cut and to lose the Oedipal struggle, to make room for absence – the same absence that is nothing but the entry ticket to the social order.

Structure and Roles in the Clinical Encounter

Much like the quaternary pattern was going to define Dora as a woman, and much like in primitive societies the pattern of relations between a woman and her brother determine that between child and its sibling, the clinic is a structure that sets the roles for those who frequent it – psychoanalyst and patient. At first sight, the clinic does not appear to represent the quaternary, because at any given moment in time, it clearly includes only two people. Yet the analogical quaternary structure nevertheless forms the background to the clinical encounter. After all, the stage is set by an earlier analyst-patient dyad – for instance Freud and his first patient, who first instituted the structure. The psychoanalyst thinks: "Like Freud to his patient, I am to mine – therefore I am a psychoanalyst!"

In this structure, the psychoanalyst occupies the role of the object, thereby assisting the patient in becoming a subject. The analyst, by staying in a silent, neutral position, and thus offering themselves to the patient's speculations about their thoughts and feelings, occupies the position of the object in subject-object relations. This positioning drives the patient into taking the position of the speaking subject who expresses themselves. If the analyst would say "they mean nothing to me" about another patient, this would harm all of her or his other patients. The statement would hold for them as well in so far as they too occupy the same role in the structure.

We may wonder whether psychoanalysts can really be neutral. Can they avoid taking the role of a desiring subject? And what does all this mean if we take into account that all analysts themselves will have been in an analysis? Having invested such an effort to attain subjecthood, must they now divest themselves of that when taking the position of an analyst? The paradox here is that psychoanalysis is also a training process in the sense of being a psychically formative experience. Subjects in analysis take part in a process that makes them more of a subject, more desirous, more in touch with their drives. What's the point of all this, if future psychoanalysts, who have finally learned to more fully embrace their subjecthood, then choose to become analysts only to find themselves occupying the object position? Could it be that the more successful their treatment is, the more they are required to forgo the fruits of this success?

But coming to occupy the subject position does not mean the end of the analysis. In psychotherapy, this might be the point at which the process is terminated, but psychoanalysis goes one step beyond subjecthood. The changes supported by the therapeutic process enable patients to grow into subjects with the ability to express and experience their desire, but this is followed by recognition that subjecthood is produced by a symbolic system. Such recognition of our being part of the structure into which we were born reduces narcissistic identification as a desired object and leads us to understand that our desire as subjects, too, is generated by myth. Now patients are willing to see themselves as subjects in a symbolic structure, who can choose to be objects. With this they can work, should they choose, to become psychoanalysts.

Analysts, during a treatment, must agree to surrender themselves (Freud 1926) in order for the structure to operate on them. They must be willing to bear the transference; the signifiers their patients attribute to them with the emotions and fantasies produced by these signifiers. In the course of analysis, the analysand recognizes how much their fate is caused by signifiers. When they accept it, they can live a desire, propelled by a story. In a similar way, the analysand who chose to be an analyst is surrendering themselves to the fate that is determined by the signifiers of the transference.

References

Ager, Sheila L. (2021). Royal brother–sister marriage, Ptolemaic and otherwise. In E. D. Carney & S. Müller (Eds.), *The Routledge Companion to Women and Monarchy in the Ancient Mediterranean World* (pp. 346–358). Routledge.

Bascom, W. R. (1969). *The Yoruba of Southwestern Nigeria*. Holt, Rinehart and Winston.

England, J. (2014). A new physics theory of life, *Quanta Magazine*, https://www.quantamagazine.org/a-new-thermodynamics-theory-of-the-origin-of-life-20140122/.

Freud, S. (1905). Fragment of an Analysis of a Case of Hysteria. In J. Strachey (Ed. and Trans.), *The standard edition of the complete psychological works of Sigmund Freud* (Vol. 7, pp. 3–123). Hogarth Press.

Freud, S. (1920). *Beyond the pleasure principle* (J. Strachey, Trans.; Standard Edition, Vol. 18, pp. 7–64). Hogarth Press.

Freud, S. (1926). *The question of lay analysis: Conversations with an impartial person*. W.W. Norton & Company.

Freud, S. (1957). Mourning and melancholia. In J. Strachey (Trans.) *The standard edition of the complete psychological works of Sigmund Freud* (Vol. 14, pp. 243–259). Hogarth Press.

Kirch, P. V. (2019). *How chiefs became kings: Divine kingship and the rise of archaic states in ancient Hawai'i*. University of California Press.

Lévi-Strauss, C. (1969). *The elementary structures of kinship* (J. H. Bell, J. R. von Sturmer, & R. Needham, Trans.). Beacon Press.

Lévi-Strauss, C. (1990). *The raw and the cooked* (J. Weightman & D. Weightman, Trans.). Harper & Row.

Voruz, V. (2007). A Lacanian reading of Dora. In *The later Lacan: An introduction* (pp. 158–179). State University of New York Press.

Chapter 5

Totemism

Yehuda Israely

Lévi-Strauss's Approach to Totemism

Totemism held a special interest for Lévi-Strauss, bringing together various aspects of the structural approach. Group identity is grounded in myths in which the totem can be observed to interact with the world. Myths articulate the tribe's singular place vis-à-vis other groups and this is represented by their respective totems. Another function of the totem is that it regulates exogamy through the taboo against marriage among group members. Though in the eyes of western anthropologists, natives' use of the totem may appear irrational, mythically presenting them as the offspring of some primeval animal, the totem also reflects advanced logical and mathematical thinking of the kind that supports complex marriage-related algorithms. But this requires "reading" the totem structurally, following Lévi-Strauss's method.

Usually, the totem consists of an animal species, taking the role of the primeval father in the tribe's mythology. As such it symbolizes the bond between the tribe's members, much like nations rally under national flags. In very abstract terms, we may say that the totem represents the domain of the symbol even before human individuals are born into it. Before the actual relations among individuals and groups emerge, there are the relations among entities with which humans identify. Myth renders the relations among tribes as relations among totems, with each totem representing a tribe. This system of symbolic relations determines that marriage is only sanctioned with members of other tribes, i.e., belonging to another totem. As a result, even before a new infant is born, constraints are in place about who she or he may marry when the time comes. Traces of such a prohibition can be observed in the practices of the Ororo tribe in Brazil, whom, as mentioned, Lévi-Strauss (1969) studied: the tribal people call "father," anyone who lawfully qualifies for paternity. Differences among anthropologists, especially the debate between structuralists and functionalists, become more pointed where totemism is concerned. Lévi-Strauss criticized his functionalist colleagues' "totemic illusion," which considered the totem testimony to the last vestiges of man's identification with animals. Natives, according to them, think of

DOI: 10.4324/9781003773764-6

themselves as animals. Structural anthropologists saw this as functionalists' own projection onto the natives. Tribal people, to them, appeared closer to animals than themselves, for instance because they believed that, say, the armadillo could have been their ancient, biological precursor. Showing that the totem is a metaphor or symbol, Lévi-Strauss proved a mechanism, squarely opposed to the functionalist assumption, whereby all myth starts off with an act of separation from the animal domain.

The work of Scottish anthropologist J. G. Frazer illustrates the kind of misunderstanding and superiority represented by functionalism. Much of Lévi-Strauss's novel approach was formulated as part of his criticism of Frazer. The solidarity that marks Lévi-Strauss's approach is essentially in reaction to Frazer's views on totemism. For Frazer, identification with an animal symbol showed traces of a time preceding the discovery of the role of the male in human fertility. Frazer took it that since they attributed a paternal role to nature, native people believed the primeval father to be non-human, a force of nature symbolized as an animal. This is how functionalism assumed native people were misguided about the world around them. Frazer believed that enlightened western people, by contrast, had left such views behind: this exactly was what it meant to be civilized. Frazer was followed by Malinowski (1929), who interpreted the sexual openness of the Trobrianders as evidence of their ignorance of male fertility. Lévi-Strauss saw this as these scholars' way of setting themselves apart from primitive people.

One of the roles of the totem, arguably, is to give shape to a community. Often taking the form of an animal, it imbues the community with life by way of this animistic image. Present-day "totems," like the donkey and elephant emblems, respectively, of the US Republican and Democratic parties, might lead us to treat them as living creatures with distinct sets of features, drives and wishes. That would be a mistake. In Lévi-Strauss's perspective, a community is not a living creature but a symbolic entity. The totem, however, holds out the animistic illusion that the community is a living creature.

The animal serving as the totemic emblem in native societies is always a type or genus of animal – as in the Talmudic verse, "The starling went to the crow for a reason" or, "Birds of a feather flock together," which is to say: two related types will look for each other. Animals in myths are deployed in an essentially different way than, say, in modern animations like Roger Rabbit or Mickey Mouse, each of which are very particular characters. The totem will never refer to the specific rabbit but to the entire genus. As such, the totem should be seen as something else than the tutelary animal acting as personal guardian, widespread in native American cultures. Such a tutelary animal may be a wolf, but the reference will be to a specific wolf – a white wolf with a black star on its forehead. The totem, rather than offering this type of individual protection, functions as a family name. It is a face for the community. In myths recounting the emergence of humans and of the tribe, the totem is central. Having symbolically generated the tribe, the totem carries the title of the tribe's archaic father. This father is no more – and no less – an actual father than the pope.

Zhuangzi's Butterfly and the Totem as Mirror Image

In the Chinese parable, Zhuangzi has a dream in which he is a butterfly. When he wakes up, he wonders: now, am I a butterfly who dreams he is Zhuangzi? Lacan (1964) believes that in this story, the butterfly features as Zhuangzi's mirror image. In the mirror stage, the child ties its identity to its image as reflected in the mirror. As an identification, this is mistaken: what the child sees is no more than an image. This image does not include the child's desires and drives. The apparent completeness of the image glosses over conflicts and absences. It seems to us that this image is us, because we crave representation. For want of better, we accept this image the mirror holds out – this face, this form. I will identify with this so I might have a shape.

The butterfly in this parable is a kind of totem, an identity-giving animal. Nothing but a representation, this totem doesn't essentially differ from the mirror image, which is a representation too. Identification with "totems" can be observed in children: when they engage in pretend games, they will "be" a rabbit now, and next they'll be a cat. Little Hans said: "I am a horse." The mirror image, or the butterfly totem – they make possible our visible existence: we emerge under the gaze. The notion of emergence under the gaze Lacan (1982) took from the French phenomenological philosopher, Maurice Merleau-Ponty, a contemporary of his. Visual representation can be flattened into a stain: it need not be the human figure in the mirror or the butterfly totem. All it needs is a stain standing out against a background. That is what it takes to stand out: the point of identification is differentiation. Likewise, the mirror image has a distinctive outline: the gaze offers both outline and consistency.

In his *Portrait of the Artist as A Young Man* (1916), James Joyce describes his protagonist, Stephen Dedalus, as a boy, writing his address: "Stephen Dedalus / Class of Elements / Clongowes Wood College / Sallins / County Kildare/ Ireland / Europe / The World / The Universe" (Joyce 1916 p. 12) – once he gets this far, he panics, dizzy with a sense of infinity. To cope, he goes on to imagine a kind of rope, wrapped around the entire universe. Humans have a need for outline. Much like Stephen Dedalus, who projected himself as far out as he could, the subject, identifying with its ego, craves circumscription. This need takes us to the very beginnings of development, to the need to identify with a mark, a spot or stain, something we may also understand as the inception of the ancient need for a totem. Freud addresses this need in "Group Psychology and the Analysis of the Ego" as one of the three identifications, hysteric identification with someone through a common desire, an identification as an object belonging to a subject, and identification through a common mark.

To revert to Zhuangzi's dream: Being Zhuangzi comes with the full weight of responsibility for what it means to carry that specific name, in his particular culture; being a butterfly, by contrast, suggests the possibility to escape from his many roles in the chain of signifiers. While the butterfly is free – we may say – Zhuangzi is captured like a butterfly in a net of signifiers. It is thanks to the signifier that the subject exists, but she or he is constrained by it, too. In psychoanalysis, we contemplate the narrative in which we live from an external vantage point. This is the liberation psychoanalysis can offer: while enabling the desire produced by the myth's signifiers, it does so at some remove, yielding up a certain distance from the signifier.

The advantage of identification with the butterfly over identification as Zhuangzi, is that the former concerns a mere act of representation, while the mirror image suggests it holds a person's essence. Where identification is regarding an entire community, the image of the body falters. The image of the body can only belong to one person. Hence, when – like a stain under the gaze – the community seeks to define itself, it reaches for a totem. Anything might have sufficed instead. But the human body, which belongs to the private individual, cannot quite be. The community will have to choose a sign of identity. Cultures will select their symbol or emblem from the living – whether animal or vegetal – world around them. What exactly they choose matters less – it is crucial that there is agreement about the totem. Say we all agree that an exclamation mark defines us then this turns us into a community. It will make little difference if, instead, we had chosen a question mark to function in this role.

Shackleton, the south pole explorer, recounted how, after their ship got stuck in ice, he and two other members of the crew went in search of a way out (Lansing 1959). Though he knew they were three, again and again, on these reconnaissance trips, he'd struggle against a feeling that another, fourth member of the group was missing. Shackleton believed this was because, thinking of the group as an entity, he couldn't stop himself from including it as another member of the group itself. This touches on paradoxes we know from mathematical group theory. Is the group itself a member of the group? Using a person as a totem for the group caused the confusion of Shackleton, counting an extra person in the group.

The basic function of the totem, therefore, is to make the group stand out as a distinct, countable entity – it is the unary sign for the group.

"Totem and Taboo" and Lévi-Straussian Kinship Relations

The word *totem* originated among the native peoples living around the great lakes of northern America. It signifies: "this person is a relative of mine". For Lévi-Strauss, in addition to offering an animistic representation of the community, the totem has three other social-organizational functions: (1) it brings together a group sharing family relations; (2) it distinguishes the own group from other groups with different totems, and (3) it generates myths about social relations between the groups. Such groups, or "clans," are somewhere along the line between what we know as extended family and tribe. A "tribe" is the more inclusive notion and can hold together a large number of totems.

In the context of kinship relations, the totem constitutes a phase in the evolution of exogamy. The next stage following the exchange of sisters and avunculate marriage, is *moiety*, which, as mentioned, refers to "halves." Now the clan is divided into two halves, which are committed to marrying only with the other half's members. This expands both the inventory of available brides and grooms, and the required social trust: if, in the past, a man could only marry one of his cousins, now any unmarried woman of the other moiety is a possible candidate. The myths that give shape to the relations between moieties will present them as opposing pairs: one will be black, the other white; one tall, the other short. This contrast makes it possible to see the joining of marital partners as an act furthering harmony and the resolution of oppositions: thesis, antithesis, and synthesis. Next comes a stage of more radical exogamy, with the emergence of the taboo: "Only not with women from your own tribe." Now there is no more positive prescription; what remains is prohibition alone. The totem is the shared symbol of a group of blood relations who are bound by sexual prohibition.

Totems are accompanied by taboos. They employ a statistical model in the sense that by determining what is prohibited, they confirm that everything else is allowed. A member of your own tribe is off limits; members of all other tribes are admissible. Taboo becomes relevant wherever it's hard to give up or forgo. Diverse cultures carry ritual representations showing how hard it is to refrain from sexual relations with first-order blood relatives as required by exogamy. The marriage ceremony of the Ifugao people of the Philippines (Lévi-Strauss 1969) starts off by mimicking war. First the tribes engage in fighting, and when it is time to make peace, women are exchanged in marriage. Circassian weddings involve the ritual ravishing of the bride. What's the reason behind this custom? It's clear the bride is willing to go with the groom – or else she would not participate in the ritual. The ritual coheres with another Circassian custom: that of the avunculate. The bride is released with some reluctance; the ravisher pays a dowry agreed by all. The ceremonial ravishing enacts the phantasm that a woman could actually stay with her father and brothers, by staging disavowal of incestuous harmony. The ceremonial fights between the moieties reveals the traces of phantasm – an earlier state of fullness.

Methods Mechanical and Statistical – What's Allowed and What Isn't

In many hunter–gatherer societies it is common to have rules such as, the hunter who aimed the first arrow that hits receives the heart of the buffalo. The one who shot the fatal arrow gets the liver. The remaining offal is distributed among the clan. There is an established division for the other parts of the animal: it is based on family connections. Brothers receive the fore legs, brothers-in-law the hind legs, and all else is divided among the rest of the clan members. No one stays hungry. This method carefully calculates each person's share. Its clear division and introduction of order parallels kinship relations. A man is obliged to marry his maternal cousin; if this is not possible, then his second- or third-order maternal cousin. The rules about which part of the body are given out to whom are very clear – whether the body is that of the killed animal or, more metaphorically, of the family.

In contrast with the above mechanical method of distribution, taboo-governed distribution is more streamlined and abstract. Rather than telling everyone what to do, it only articulates from what to abstain; all else is allowed by implication. Jewish as well as Islamic ritual food laws are taboo based. An Amazonian hunter-gatherer's tribe are allowed to eat all animals, but the men must refrain from eating the meat of the opossum, associated with maternity because the female opossum carries its cubs on her back.

Cultures can be distinguished in terms of their tendency towards either a "mechanistic" or "statistical" semanticity, something that will be reflected in a variety of cultural expressions and behaviors. It will be manifest in all of the culture's idioms – not just in the way people talk and write, but equally in the way they cook or make music – as well as, of course, in how they marry. The "mechanistic" nature of a society like China, which comes under the Sino-Tibetan language family, is reflected both in how people speak and how they get married: synonyms are relatively rare, and there is no abundance of alternative brides and grooms. There is one correct choice. The Indo-European language family, by contrast, has a more "statistical" or open style. One word may, depending on context, have a range of meanings, and languages offer a choice of synonyms. The totemic method I discussed above is statistical in nature and relies on taboo. Except for what is prohibited, do what you want.

Taboo Unfolding – From Source of Pleasure to Prohibition, and From Home Out into the World

One way of thinking about the phenomenon of taboo is to observe how what began as a source of sensual pleasure eventually transformed into a prohibited act. The Maranganji aboriginals in Australia tell a myth in which, long ago, the one food available to the people was the totem animal; today it is the only thing they are forbidden to consume. This appears to run parallel with the present prohibition on sexual intercourse and marriage with the tribe's women, who once were the only source of sexual pleasure. The same can be observed on the level of individual infant development, where the mother initially is the one single source of erotic satisfaction. In time, both she and the male child's sisters become an object of grave prohibition. The prohibition on consuming the totemic animal, in fact, can also be seen as a version of the prohibition on incest. Delayed gratification, and the injunction to refrain from what was, to begin with, a main source of pleasure, is a very frequent motif. This is reflected not only in rules directly addressing sexuality but also involves actions and objects that metaphorically stand for sexuality – first and foremost, eating (Lévi-Strauss 1972).

Among the Akan people of the Ivory Coast, the word *nkom* refers to both eating and getting married at the same time. The Australian Kuku-Yalanji people use one and the same word – *ardan* – to denote cannibalism and incest. Language reflects the degree to which delayed gratification pervades a culture's different domains, with each functioning as a metaphor for the others. In our own culture, too, we call a sexually violent person a "predator" – a term deriving from the animal kingdom. New Guinea's Arapesh people (Lévi-Strauss 1969), have an extremely clear and blunt formulation staking out the prohibition on one's own and access to anything that isn't, in a sentence that manifests a similar attitude to delayed gratification in divergent domains: "Your mother, your sister, your pigs, the pile of yams that you have stacked with your own hands – all of these you are forbidden to eat. The mothers of other people, the sisters of other people, the pigs of other people, the piles of yams that others have stacked – you are allowed to eat." The taboo on using certain personally owned resources, and the corresponding need to exchange resources with other groups, drives a culture to forge connections with others. In certain restaurants in rural France, there is a custom whereby one drinks one's neighbor's wine. You bring your own wine, and others bring theirs, and each drinks the other's wine. People become friends in this way. All it takes is to taste from a stranger's wine – once you take a sip, you're no longer strangers. Kindergarten children in China wear pinafores that are tied from behind: as a result, the children have to help each other – a sure way to inculcate cooperation.

Back to Freud's "Totem and Taboo"

Here is a myth from New Guinea's Yafar tribe: a son is building a hut but doesn't manage to get in place its chief support. His mother tells him to ask for help from his father. The father descends into the building pit where the pillar is supposed to be secured. He lies belly down on the ground, telling his son to drive the pillar through his back. Thus, he gives his own body, his flesh, to support the new home of his son (Juillot 1962). This myth has an Oedipal dimension: the mother helps her son by sacrificing the father's life. But unlike Freud's classical Oedipal scenario where the son kills the father – here the father volunteers to die. Death, in the idiom of myth means negation or denial, sacrificing the concrete or real in exchange for the symbolic. Here this substitution takes the shape of replacing the father with a hut. It reveals Lévi-Strauss's view of the totem as representative of the community, whose core is the family – symbolized in this myth by the hut.

In Lacanian interpretations Freud and Lévi-Strauss are brought together. The function of the Oedipal father who puts himself between child and mother is the function of the father as the law of exogamy. Lacan takes the father signifier to an even more radical place by turning it into the linchpin of the symbolic order. For him, the signifier "name of the father" validates the claim of a collection of signs to be a structure of signifiers, thereby transforming noises into meaningful words.

So, which of the two principles – exogamy or the Oedipus – is the more crucial cultural condition? This is the debate between the two respective theoretical approaches and to gain a better grip on it, let's consider the place of the totem in that conversation. For Freud, in "Totem and Taboo" (1912–1913), the totem serves to solve Oedipal aggression aimed at the father. The clinical description of little Hans's phobia offers an instance of Oedipal-totemic interpretation. Here the figure of the horse features as a substitute for the father as target of fear and aggression. Lévi-Strauss, by contrast, considers the totem in relation to exogamy: totemism comes to organize kinship relations and marriage rules between clans, rather than arranging things within the nuclear family. These two models differ mainly because they have different objectives. While Oedipal relations define intergenerational configurations in traditional families, parents and children – exogamy structures relations between equals: siblings, or community members.

There are two key laws of the totem: the totemic animal must not be killed, and the women who come under the totem are sexually out of bounds. The upshot is that the totem defines a certain group – usually a tribe or part of a tribe – whose women are taboo for the men of the tribe. The connection with Freud is not hard to observe: the prohibition on killing the totemic animal and the taboo on the women belonging under the same totem is tantamount to declaring that one mustn't kill one's father or have sex with one's mother. But Lévi-Strauss understands this differently: the totem represents all of the tribe's men who compete over the family's women. Freud's and Lévi-Strauss's methods may turn out to clash less than would appear if we understand Freud's interpretation in "Totem and Taboo" to suggest that competition with all males, in general, can be traced back to that between father and son.

Lévi-Strauss argued there is no need for an archetypical father-son relationship underlying all male competition for there to be such competition and, hence, the law of exogamy. He believed that Freud took insufficient account of how the family system was related to that of clan and society. In the same vein, he disagreed with Radcliffe-Brown (1952), the anthropologist who, like Freud, took mother-father-child as the basic family unit, with the rest of the clan taking a secondary place. Radcliffe-Brown drew a line between the nuclear family and the social system. For Lévi-Strauss both critically failed to observe continuities between these two levels, the micro and the macro.

Lacan's position, as mentioned, helps to bridge here. For him the source of competition in human experience is neither Oedipal nor totemic, but rather the imaginary stage that forms the root of both family and society. The child competes with its mirror image, which appears completer and more lovable than itself. The child itself too falls victim to its charms. This, for Lacan, is where both Oedipal strife and contestations around the tribe's women, originate. Lévi-Strauss's siblings, much like Freud's fathers, join the antagonist's position only later. The double, in Lacan's mirror image, preceded them. Lacan's perspective settles the difference between Freud and Lévi-Strauss, by presenting it as a splitting caused by the aggressive, imaginary drive. It is, then, left to the symbolic law of the father – whether in the form of the totem or the father of the family.

Freud's Personal Blind Spot

For Lévi-Strauss the maternal uncle is part of the fundamental family structure, which cannot exist without including and connecting with some other entities. Small family units must connect to each other and into a community, and therefore exogamy is key to the family. A metaphor from physics can illustrate this; a molecule consists of a number of interconnected atoms. It's the electrons they share that link among these atoms. We can liken the role of the uncle to that of the electron: while part of the atom's basic cell, it also serves to connect between different atoms. The uncle belongs to both his sister's and his wife's families. Why did Freud "overlook" relationships within the community?

We might want to say that here we have a blind spot, marking the limits of Freud's self-analysis. A possible explanation for this lack of insight lies in his personal life. Having married Martha Bernays, sister of Eli Bernays who married Freud's own sister, Anna, Freud in fact lived the fundamental exogamic scenario.

Lévi-Strauss observed how difficult it is to analyze the myths by which we live ourselves. He saw this as the reason for the arrogance of earlier anthropologists: they ignored the myths by which they lived – which were myths, nevertheless, however little they might resemble those of tribal cultures. About himself, he said – with some envy – that he could not be affected by the magical influence of native myths (Lévi-Strauss 1962) because he was not part of their mythologies. And regarding the myths to which he belonged, such as "academia" or "anthropology," he admitted his analytic faculty was severely limited. The consoling, unifying and inclusive function of myth clashes with the analytical function needed to decipher its workings. Telling the story while also living it at the same time is a tall order. It's hard to laugh at a joke when you have to explain it. To further illustrate the clash between the position of observer and that of the one who is situated within the experience Lévi-Strauss recounted how he tended not to remember what he had written. Writing escaped him, as it were, in a flow of creative energy, immersed in the myth of structural theory.

As we explore these traditional frameworks, it's important to recognize the evolving nature of family structures in today's society. Modern families often extend beyond traditional definitions, incorporating diverse and fluid configurations that reflect broader societal changes. This evolution challenges us to draw insights from both Oedipal and exogamic models while understanding their limitations in capturing the full spectrum of modern relationships.

The task is to integrate these historical perspectives with an awareness of contemporary dynamics, where family roles and relationships are increasingly shaped by choice and mutual respect rather than fixed hierarchies. This shift encourages us to rethink how we interpret kinship and relational dynamics, fostering a dialogue that respects the varied experiences and identities within families today.

References

Freud, S. (1912–1913). Totem and taboo. In J. Stracheyet *al.* (Trans.), *The standard edition of the complete psychological works of Sigmund Freud,* Volume XIII. Hogarth Press.

Joyce, J. (1916). *A portrait of the artist as a young man.* B. W. Huebsch.

Juillot, B. (1962). *La pensée sauvage.* Gallimard.

Lacan, J. (1964). *The seminar of Jacques Lacan: Book IX: The identification (1961–1962)* (G. Hamilton, Trans.). W. W. Norton & Company.

Lacan, J. (1982). *The seminar of Jacques Lacan: Book XI: The four fundamental concepts of psychoanalysis (1963–1964)* (J. Miller, Trans.). W. W. Norton & Company.

Lansing, A. (1959). *Endurance: Shackleton's incredible voyage.* McGraw-Hill Book Company.

Lévi-Strauss, C. (1962). *La pensée sauvage.* Gallimard.

Lévi-Strauss, C. (1969). *The elementary structures of kinship* (J. H. Bell, J. R. von Sturmer, & R. Needham, Trans.). Beacon Press.

Lévi-Strauss, C. (1972). *The savage mind* (G. Weidenfeld & Nicolson Ltd., Trans.). University of Chicago Press. (Original work published 1962.)

Malinowski, B. (1929). *The sexual life of savages in north-western Melanesia.* Routledge.

Radcliffe-Brown, A. R. (1952). *Structure and function in primitive society.* Routledge & Kegan Paul.

Chapter 6

Myth

Yehuda Israely

Of all the domains in which Lévi-Strauss worked, myth comes closest to our own sphere of interest as psychoanalysts. Almost everything patients say in the clinic can be seen as myth and, consequently, can be structurally analyzed.

Myth as Carrier of Existential Contradictions

Lévi-Strauss (1963) defines myth as a system of signifiers whose function is to allow the coexistence of existential contradictions This definition resembles Freud's definition of psychoanalytic work. When the psychoanalyst seeks to resolve repression, it is not with the aim of resolving conflict but rather to make that conflict conscious. The idea behind this is that the symptom represents unconscious conflict, and in so far as this conflict becomes conscious, or rather: to the extent it is put into words – the symptom, which represented the conflict, becomes dispensable.

Like psychoanalysis, myth seeks to solve – within the domain of language – problems that are the outcome of our being speaking creatures. Myths tend on the whole to touch upon universal topics like birth, death, or sexuality. They emerge around existential conflicts that have no resolution in reality. We will have to manage with the fact that humans, as symbolic creatures, are conflicted and torn, but myths can make it easier.

Myths can help us cope with these intolerable existential contradictions by comparing them, metaphorically, with a story in which a solution is achieved. Death, for instance, is something we find hard to accept – it is, one might say, one of the existential problems with which humanity struggles and it has no solution. Poems, however, do offer solutions. For example, the idiom "mother earth" can be a solution to the fear of death, making death and burial a return to the mother. The clash between the joy of living and the fear of death may be settled if "returning to dust" is the same as "returning to a mother's arms." We are presented with an analogy between the child returning to their mother, and the human being who is made of dust and eventually returns to dust. The gap between the living person and their death – a and b – is like that between a son and his mother – c and d,

DOI: 10.4324/9781003773764-7

and, as a result, when the living go to their death, it is like children returning to their mother.

To create an effect of resolution, the contradiction one seeks to resolve in vain is compared with another contradiction that does have a solution and with which the possibility of reconciliation exists. The first contradiction, between life and death, is represented metaphorically in the second contradiction, between leaving the mother's body at birth and returning to her in death. If the earth is the mother, then there is no clash between where life versus where death takes us. All of this aligns with how meaning essentially emerges through a contrast between analogies. To say that contradiction A is like contradiction B is to imply that if contradiction B can be solved, then contradiction A, too, allows for resolution. Here, then, is a clinical illustration of how an analogy between one insufferable conflict and another that can be tolerated may take the edge off an existential fact that is too hard to contain. I attended a case presentation concerning a patient who had lost her husband and had a very hard time moving on with her own life. How was this experience of stuckness in the face of loss resolved? It happened when, in a meeting with her therapist, she referred to her deceased husband, with a slip of the tongue, as "my former husband." In doing so the patient drew an analogy between death and divorce. The effect was that meanings related to divorce were, through the analogy, poured into intolerable widowhood – the main one of which, perhaps, would be that after divorcing it is not only legitimate, but maybe even necessary, to move on. Additional meanings that might have transferred from divorce into widowhood, were, that divorce is not as absolute as death, or that it involves a degree of mutuality – she, equally, separates from him. Sudden death does not allow a process of separation, and the analogy with divorce which does usually include such a process, enabled this patient to reposition herself in relation to the loss of her husband.

Before starting a treatment – whether from the patient's own, or the therapist's, position – the patient's condition, as presented, may seem quite desperate. How are we to change the past? Isn't that impossible? Isn't the past irreversible – set in stone? But the more aware we are that we live by myths, the freer we are to change our history. Or rather, to change our perception of that history and the story we tell about it, and as a result, the way we experience it as well. It was the analogy between death and divorce that soothed the widow.

Myth and History – in Culture and in the Clinic

We can look at the stories circulating in a culture, much like those more personal ones brought into the clinic, as histories as well as myths. Historical interpretations will tend to assume that concrete and random events influence people and cause them to evolve in a certain way. Mythic interpretation will argue that events rather than being random, are part of a narrative plot.

Where this type of interpretation is used, events are registered with hindsight, after being adjusted to the myth's template. Psychoanalysis addresses the random: "This or that is how you are because some things happen to have occurred around you at the time of your birth, and even more so: because certain words were said which got themselves engraved upon your mind." An abundance of possible mythic interpretations, producing infinite chains of meanings, burdens the patient. "If this is what happened, that means that… which in turns means…" and so on. Historical interpretation, which does not hold out meanings, brings metonymic slippage to a halt, by meeting the question of "Why?" with the simple reply "Because." This, anyway, is the way to work with neurotic patients who are so overwhelmed by the self-mythologies within which they live. A patient may, for instance, wonder repeatedly why he does not like to receive compliments: what purpose could this serve in his life? He piles up interpretations, say, to the effect that it must be about him shying away from taking up space, or that he takes pride in his own modesty. But these explanations remain unsatisfactory, so he keeps inventing more. The explanations share one theme, namely, that he, the patient, is "not OK." They are psychological myths whose role it is to make sense of his psychic experience. Alternatively, these meanings may be reduced to the following statement: "This is the reality into which I was born. I have a brother with special needs, and I learned how to avoid raising his envy. How come I have a brother like that? I just did." With psychotic patients, though, the work may be in the opposite direction: we will want to include them in the common myths by which people live, so they may participate in the community and share its meanings.

How about cultural heritage? Lévi-Strauss (1981) refers to the cultural and discursive status of the French Revolution as an example of how a story can feature as both history and myth at one and the same time. Though we naturally tend to think about the French Revolution as history, while assuming that myth's role is to produce meaning, the French Revolution as a story also underwrites the meaning of democracy. So, when the story of the French revolution is cited by a politician who inflects it in discussing currently burning issues, then despite having an historical, diachronic aspect, here the story is brought to bear due to its mythic, synchronous aspect – its relevance right now. As if the French Revolution were happening in the present each time it is mentioned.

In oral cultures, before writing was invented, knowledge was held in the narrative, the spoken word. The historical narrative is diachronic and one-directional. Earlier events affect the meaning of later ones. And the same goes for the order of the words telling the historical story: it is diachronic, with one following the other in sequence. Myth, as opposed to diachronic history, is synchronous and timeless. Here future events, too, can affect the meaning of earlier ones. Though the story of the myth may be told in linear sequence, one word after the other, its structure, rather than being linear is multi-dimensional.

We get some idea of this multi-dimensionality when we look at a myth's many different versions. Since dreams share the multi-dimensionality of myth, we do not attach value to the order of events in them. Rather than approaching the signifiers in a linear mode we will treat them as fundamentally scattered.

In our clinical work we shall have to ask ourselves when to focus on the historical side of an interpretation, and when on the mythical. A therapist may for instance realize a regular pattern: her patient keeps shifting this way and that, indecisively. This back-and-forth motion appears again and again; in a variety of situations the patient describes: each time he nearly makes a decision and then pulls out again. During one session, the patient seems to recollect a relevant event from his childhood but next he reports that the memory escapes him, then again it nearly surfaces, only once more to withdraw and disappear. Because the therapist chooses to relate to the myth rather than the narrative, rather than joining the patient in his vein attempt at capturing the elusive childhood memory and in the symptomatic game, she instead reflects on the phenomenon or myth of "back and forth" which he inhabits. Rather than commenting, "Let's try for some associations to help you capture the lost memory," she observes, "There it is again: this movement back and forth."

When we are not sure whether to take an historical or a mythic perspective vis-à-vis a patient's story, we should be careful to avoid offering symbolic-mythic interpretations. This is especially relevant in the case of post-trauma, where the patient might be presenting with actual, historical memories. A patient's materials include both historical and mythic elements – at one and the same time. Though these may be events that took place in the past, they are told time and time again because they underwrite a certain meaning. Dreams utilize the remainders of a day's events to tell a story that rehearses a meaning. In the same way, symptoms can both constitute a statement and a memory, simultaneously.

Symptom and myth are related. We explained that myth's role is to make life's conflicts and contradictions more bearable: symptoms are the way in which the unconscious, notwithstanding repression, informs us about inner conflict. Often, being able to tell the story, and constructing a myth that enables living to the side of conflict makes a symptom redundant and helps it disappear. The psychic problems suffered by soldiers who serve in an occupying army are symptoms aimed at relieving conflicts when no myth is available. In 1986, during Israel's First Lebanon War, the film "Two Fingers from Sidon" was released in the cinemas. The film is about soldiers' moral dilemmas amid a captured civilian population. The film did not present solutions to the conflict – it only made it visible. Myth displays contradictions rather than blurring them, and the film, by functioning as a type of local myth, allowed the viewers to experience these contradictions.

Rather confusingly, this film was produced by the Israeli army itself. We would not expect the IDF to expose both soldiers and the Israeli public at large to the moral dilemmas of which it itself is the cause. In fact, the film was intended to be shown to higher-ranking officers only, aiming to give them a better insight into their soldiers' moral-psychological issues. When the film eventually found its way to the general public, there was an outcry among Knesset members who objected to this exposure, which they believed might undermine the army's operational capacities. The Army Spokesperson defended the choice by arguing that it would help reduce post-trauma and help soldiers execute their military missions. Soldiers, they explained, who experience conflicts without being helped to give vent to their emotions, suffer from seriously compromised, and sometimes even endangered mental health. The point of the film was to allow them to live with these conflicts without resorting to taking only one side. To contain the conflicting identifications.

Similarly, it is the role of the psychoanalyst, rather than resolving conflicts, to make them visible to reduce the damage done by repression, and the subsequent emergence of symptoms. Couple therapy is a good case in point because it seeks to lead both partners to recognize the conflict; it aims for each partner to acknowledge the other's unmet desires, without rushing to fulfil the need. Often this alone is enough, and the need to "resolve" the couple's actual conflict disappears. Once they are willing to listen to, and understand each other, they will be able to endure the conflict without it turning into a symptom, like interminable quarrels.

What Freud Thought About Myth – Psychoanalytic Treatment as Construction of Functional Myths

Unlike Plato and Aristotle, who saw popular myth, and even Greek mythology, as irrational nonsense, Freud believed that cultural myths were just as important as the personal myths that take the shape of dreams or symptoms. For him, these cultural myths were nothing but forms of organized knowledge, a type of "delusion," or recipe for dealing with human relations. The psychotic person's problem is not that they suffer from delusional thinking but the fact that their delusion happens not to be socially shared.

Freud believed the psychoanalyst's analytic work, too, participates in myth. For him, the myth evolving in the course of psychoanalytic treatment is a construction: the re-construction of the thing that might have happened in childhood. In the case of the Wolf Man, Freud achieves this by searching for the roots of some signifiers appearing in the dream, including wolves and the Roman numeral V. This leads him to conclude that the problem is trauma involving the primal scene, i.e., parental intercourse (Freud [1918] 1953). With typical intellectual integrity, Freud asks himself questions interlocutors may come up with: How can he know this? Maybe he is wrong? His answer is that while he might be mistaken, what matters is whether his explanation works. In other words, Freud acknowledges that psychoanalytic interpretation, too, is myth, but this myth has the capacity to remove the symptom, and it does so by paving the way to living alongside the conflict. Comparing the analytic myth which develops as part of the therapy with the Wolf Man's delusional myth, Freud explains that the difference between psychoanalytic delusion and psychotic delusion is that the psychotic person has no one to share with. The difference seems small, but it's crucial. In putting it this way, Freud humanizes the psychotic patient: the latter is not all that alien. We all, including the psychotic patient, have the ability to make stories and live by them. The other thing Freud's statement conveys is that we cannot but make these stories. Freud's comparison also includes an element of modesty as far as the work of the psychoanalyst is concerned: modesty and creativity. In Freud's associating between delusion or myth, and psychoanalysis, we witness the first signs of the typical postmodern awareness that we live in a symbolic and creative myth.

The Myth of the Three Caskets According to Freud

When we listen with an "ear for myth" we will be listening for mythemes: i.e., myth's minimal units of meaning, as Lévi-Strauss defined them. In the classical mythic story, the motif is fixed, while signifiers replace one another, and versions change. When we listen to a poem, we pay attention to the signifiers' sounds, meter, rhyme, and phonemic resonance. This is why it is so hard to translate poetry. Signifiers change in translation. From this point of view, mythic listening is the inverse of poetic listening. Myth lets itself be translated very easily into any existing language – even into languages that are not spoken, such as animation or dance. Its basic units consisting of motifs and myths can be translated with wide variance from the source and still preserve its meaning.

In our clinical work we must attend to the patient on the levels of the phoneme, the signifier, and the motif or mytheme simultaneously. Here is a patient recounting a dream: "I cut my pinky with a paper knife and put it in my pocket." In terms of the phoneme, we notice the repeated use of the letter -p, suggesting "penis"; in terms of the signifier – the pinky finger signifies a bodily member; in terms of the mytheme, the statement is a variation on images of castration. We must listen with three ears at the same time; we must know when one ear should pay special attention; and we must take note when these three different ears communicate one and the same message, as in this illustration.

In Shakespeare's "Merchant of Venice" the foreign suitors vie for Portia's hand. They must choose from three caskets: one made of gold, one silver, and one lead. Freud (1913) analyzes this scene, explaining that these caskets stand for types of women. Earlier versions of the same myth show this explicitly.

A major variant of the myth appears in Shakespeare's "King Lear." Here, the three caskets have transformed into the king's three daughters. Cordelia is the modest, quiet, and less striking one among them. Like the simple, duller looking metal – lead – she is the right choice in terms of the values the play champions.

The figure of Psyche, in Greek mythology is another instance: in Apuleius' myth, she is the youngest of three sisters, and Cinderella (in one of the myth's better known later versions, by the brothers Grimm) is another iteration of the third, "simple," sister. Cinderella finishes her chores aided by doves, and this enables her to be on time for the ball. Psyche similarly is helped by small animals when facing Aphrodite's test: ants come to her aid in sorting the seeds. These motifs traverse centuries, repeating the same lesson again and again: simplicity is the right way to go.

Lévi-Strauss's systemic approach assumes that myth evolves as communities share mythemes like they share genes. As in genetic evolution, "mutations" occur with every exchange between communities, whether as a result of intergenerational transmission or due to geographical proximity. While the versions grow ever more divergent, and the myth's elements undergo constant change, something remains stable: the relations between the elements. And this is exactly the great discovery of structural anthropology, offering access to the meaning of myths.

Freud, like Lévi-Strauss, sought to draw attention to how myths leach and change yet maintain a more or less stable message. To illustrate this, he referred to the myth of the three caskets (Freud 1913). If we want to make sense of ostensibly incomprehensible symptoms, he argued, we must shift our attention away from the meaning or identity of their signifiers and focus on their interrelations.

But let us return to the three caskets. Freud's reading of the "The Merchant of Venice" is that, hidden behind signifiers such as "little," "modest," "beautiful," and especially, "quiet," the play's central mytheme is death. Death, here, is represented by silence.

Freud interprets the tendency to prefer silver and gold over lead, and the two more striking, flattering girls over the sincere and simple one, as the wish to deny death. This mytheme appears across the myth's variants: now as three caskets, then as three young women, but behind these, consistently, we find the representation of death, humans' relations with it. King Lear does not want to know he is dying as a result he rejects his third daughter, the one, in this story, who represents death. Cordelia's modesty symbolizes our recognition of mortality.

In "King Lear," Cordelia eventually dies, and the old king carries off her dead body. This is the crux of tragedy: the recognition of death and finitude. The end of the play presents us with calm reconciliation to the fact that we are only mortals, not gods. This, to shift back to the clinic, is also a version of the objective of therapy: acceptance of lack. Unlike Greek tragedy, where it is death that must be accepted, in psychoanalysis death is only one form of lack or absence. Sexual difference, as it manifests in hysteria, is another instance. But the most abstract and general shape lack takes – and it can be projected onto very many representations – is the gap between word and thing: the fact that not everything can be put into words.

The motif of the choice between the three caskets renders a pseudo-choice, or rather: it presents the choice whereby we reconcile ourselves with the fact of there being no choice. There's no way around it: we all die in the end. That's what psychoanalysis is about. It dwells less on our faltering in the face of the choices we must make and more on learning to accept that it's not up to us: inevitable death, or the history into which we were born. It is our choice to stop resisting. King Lear is destined to die. The question – or his choice – is whether he will resist the death his ostensibly unappealing daughter represents.

What does the audience watching "King Lear" identify with? On the more explicit, conscious level, the play carries a moral warning against the seductions of flattery. It also elicits identification with Lear's pain at his other two daughters' ingratitude, as well as with the injustice Cordelia suffers. But Freud argues there is more to the play. King Lear is dying, yet he vainly seeks to establish who of his three daughters loves him best, as if he will live forever. He refuses to die. Carrying Cordelia's corpse in his arms, he carries death. She embodies the goddess of death who counsels the old man to give up on love. She counsels him to become reconciled with death and its inevitability.

King Lear makes regular appearances in the clinic. One of them occurs when a patient's refusal to accept death leads him to suffer from hypochondria. The need to recognize this limitation doesn't stop asserting itself. Unable to accept his mortality, his anxieties mount. He takes medication against these anxieties, but this also takes its toll as he becomes sleepy and less productive. Every experience of distress in this chain is another version of the myth about fundamental lack. This is why the psychoanalyst offers the patient interpretations, not of its specific manifestations, but of the myth itself – our refusal of imperfection.

Lacan and Myth: "The Non-Duped Err," Agreeing to Live in Myth

Lacan saw Freud's symbolic approach, which he famously summarized in the statement "the unconscious is structured like a language," (Lacan 1993 p. 119) as something precious which had to be protected from the neo-Freudians. As for Lévi-Strauss's complete perspective on the symbolic, Lacan adopted it nearly wholesale. Neither Freud nor Lévi-Strauss, however, addressed the Real in anything like Lacan's way. Freud (1930) admitted that "oceanic experience" was alien to him, while Lévi-Strauss stayed within the confines of the structuralist study of cultures. Lacan was interested in the Real – that which can be attributed neither meaning nor form and remains outside language so that any attempt to capture it in words removes it from itself. If psychoanalysis is about coming to acknowledge lack, this is the specific lack it addresses: not everything can be covered by language.

In Lacan's view, this is precisely what myth does: it seeks to capture the Real through its ever-changing variants. As no version succeeds at this, more and more narratives pile up. Wittgenstein (1954) introduced the image whereby we use words by way of a ladder that keeps us getting closer to beyond-words. For Lacan, as for Wittgenstein, the ladder is endless. This endlessness in psychotherapy takes the form of processing: the patient tells one version and then another and another of the events, in an asymptotic attempt to approach the thing itself – i.e., it is never actually reached. When Lacan states that the Real is the impossible, he is thinking of the impossibility of catching the Real by means of the Symbolical, of the epistemological tragedy in which the Real forever continues to elude us. The Real is the hypothetical core of myth, which will presumably be revealed at the end of time, after our attempts at infinite number of variants. This also explains why it is possible to exist within myth even though we know that it is only that and not the Real. When we recognize, with or without analysis, that there is no other way of being. Lacan dedicated his 1973–1974 seminar to this: "Les non-dupes errent"– a homophone of "le nom du père" ["the name of the father"]. *It is a mistake* ("errent") *to insist not to be fooled.* As a result, the cynic, who declines to play along by living in myth, finds themselves outside life. One outcome of psychoanalysis is the recognition that there is no alternative symbolic home. Before setting out on analysis, we might still believe that once all delusions and myths are abolished, we will, finally, live in truth. At the end of analysis, we realize that truth resides within myth. Truth is something we say. Truth consists of words: it is never the thing itself. What renders myth truthful in spite of this, is that it has actual effects, as we saw for instance in the myth of the romantic fit between Scorpio and Pisces, which offers any couple who takes an interest in, and believes the myth of, astrology, a real advantage in the early stages of a relationship.

In psychotherapy with neurotic patients, one of the key objectives is to agree to live in the story. Obsessive disorders are marked by the centrality of the patient's denial of the myth. The obsessive subject says: I refuse to accept and identify with the signifier. I refuse to accept that my work be labelled as a profession through which I am defined and constrained. What psychoanalysts would like to communicate to the obsessive patient is that myth is not real enough to warrant refusal. In other words: I agree with you that we're only talking about signifiers, but do you agree with yourself that it's *only* a matter of signifiers? You refuse to have anything to do with these signifiers, as if you believe they have huge power, as if they were real. But wasn't it you yourself, in the first place, who endorsed the signifier and granted it this power? Psychoanalysis strives to enable the obsessive patient to join and live in the story while recognizing it as "just a story".

In the case of hysteria, the process is similar, but instead of resisting the dubious validity of signifiers, the hysteric resists a particular person, usually an authority figure, who is perceived as an agent of the symbolic world. Here too, the patient can be offered an interpretation: the good news – it is possible to stop resisting; and the bad news – it is possible to stop resisting because there is no truly authoritative figure capable of making the signifier real.

Psychotic patients, by contrast, have difficulty experiencing themselves as part of any common, shared myth, and hence they live delusionally in private myth. Unlike obsessive subjects who, while refusing to belong, nevertheless do belong in spite of themselves, psychotic subjects lack the mental component which likens signifier to real – something which Lacan named "the name of the Father". In the case of psychotic patients, therapy aims to help them join the myth by means of the "sinthome." A sinthome can be a religion, ideology, faith, or any other narrative in which people with a psychotic psychic structure can join to feel that they have a role in the world, that they have something to contribute and have a purpose. It is a myth they can adopt, in addition to the existing structure of signifiers.

References

Freud, S. (1913). The theme of the three caskets. *The standard edition of the complete psychological works of Sigmund Freud* (Vol. 12, pp. 289–302). Hogarth Press.

Freud, S. ([1918] 1953). The wolf-man. In J. Strachey (Ed.), *The standard edition of the complete psychological works of Sigmund Freud* (Vol. 18, pp. 1–237). Hogarth Press.

Freud, S (1930). *Civilization and its discontent.* H. SE (Vol 21 pp. 421–506). Horath Press.

Lacan, J. (1973–1974). *Seminar XXI - Les Non Dupes Errent* (C. Gallagher, Trans.) Unpublished manuscript.

Lacan, J. (1993). *The seminar of Jacques Lacan, Book III: The psychoses, 1955–1956* (R. Grigg, Trans.). W. W. Norton.

Lévi-Strauss, C. (1963). Myth and meaning. In *Structural anthropology* (pp. 207–236). Basic Books.

Lévi-Strauss, C. (1981). *The origin of table manners: From the primitive to the civilized.* University of Chicago Press.

Wittgenstein, L. (1954). *Philosophical investigations.* Basil Blackwell.

Chapter 7

Psychoanalysis' Myth of Creation

Yehuda Israely

Not every myth is a myth of creation. Creation myths aim to explain the origins and order of things, humans, nature through cosmogonic narratives, but in addition, they also serve to create a reality, as in the case of the myth of the French Revolution inaugurating modern France's political reality. How did psychoanalysis come about? What is its constitutive, symbolic event? What was the creative act which, once formulated as a narrative, became a myth of creation? It was Freud's dream about Irma's injection that turned out to be the foundational moment of psychoanalysis.

The Dream about Irma's Injection: Freud's "Specimen Dream"

Freud recounts this dream in his *The Interpretation of Dreams* (1900): Referring to it as his "specimen dream" he mentioned it on several occasions in his writings. It was his dream about Irma that led him to formulate the hypothesis that dreams render the fulfilment of a wish. The wish fulfilled in his dream about Irma, he explained, was about ridding himself of his guilt for having made a mistake in his treatment of Irma, his analysand, who continued suffering from several symptoms after having been in analysis with Freud.

Birth and Birth Certificate

Freud viewed his interpretation of his dream about Irma's injection as the foundational moment of psychoanalysis. Here, he argued, was where the unconscious first manifested itself to him. He interpreted his own unconscious motivations in this dream and as it were "caught himself" producing excuses aimed to relieve him of his therapeutic responsibility. The dream about Irma's injection brought him the crucial insight that something, here, was at work, some unconscious function trying to tell a story with which his conscience could live in peace. Agreeing to remove repression, his unconscious revealed itself to him so that he could observe his own motivation, which was to prove himself innocent in the face of Irma's complaints; thereby installing not only

DOI: 10.4324/9781003773764-8

the observed unconscious but the observing analyst who was founded in the revelation. We can say that the founding act of psychoanalysis and psychoanalyst took the form of a revelation of the unconscious of the object "Freud" and the emergence of a psychoanalyst subject "Freud."

In a letter to his friend, Wilhelm Fliess, Freud wrote that one day, a plaque near his house would announce that at this site, and on this particular date, psychoanalysis was born when the secret of the unconscious was revealed to Dr Freud. The imaginary act of attaching the plaque signals the birth of a myth. We are so accustomed to the metaphor of society as a human body that we tend to forget that society neither has a body nor enjoys the pleasures of the body. There is no physical event like birth or physical state like satisfaction. This is why we have to announce an "event" by putting up a sign or plaque to render a symbolic creation present. Because society is not a body. A metaphor needs to be elaborated like putting up a plaque in space and time.

This is also where we can situate the limit of structural anthropology's potential contribution to psychoanalysis. Structural anthropology can only teach us about the Symbolic, while human beings are much more than that; they are Real.

When a human organism comes into the world, the state issues a birth certificate serving as bureaucratic confirmation of their existence. While during birth, an actual body is born, the birth certificate puts a signifier to that body. But in the case of a symbolic birth, the emergence of the symbol equals birth. There is only birth by certificate. A myth of creation is birth through certification, and in our present context, the dream about Irma's injection is psychoanalysis' "birth certificate." Only a certificate, since this is all about a symbolic event.

Lacan's Interpretation of the Dream about Irma's Injection – We Are the Addressees

Lacan also considered the dream about Irma's injection important and dedicated a profound analysis to it. He took Freud's statement that the dream constituted the founding act of psychoanalysis as his main perspective in analyzing the dream. In approaching Freud's dream – as indeed we would with any other dream – it must be treated as two simultaneous actions: that of dreaming the dream and that of interpreting it. Over and beyond interpreting the dream itself, Lacan also analyzes Freud's very choice to analyze this dream as well as his particular interpretative angle. We, Freud's students, psychoanalysts as well as anthropologists, are the addressees, he claims, of both the dream and Freud's interpretation of it. For Lacan, then, Freud had us in mind already when he was dreaming it, and next, in his analysis.

Freud's own conclusion, after analyzing his dream about Irma, was, as we've seen, that dreams are wish fulfilment. The wish, in this case, was to free himself of responsibility for having failed in Irma's treatment. Freud explains that the dream takes the form of a bunch of pretexts and explanations that all come to serve this one purpose, rather ridiculously piling them up. He compares this with what he calls "kettle logic," when a man who returns a borrowed kettle to its owners, explains the hole in it by piling up three clashing explanations: "I returned it whole"; "It had a hole in it in the first place," and "I never borrowed it." While each explanation might be reasonable in its own right, when offered together, the result cannot but sound ridiculous and suspicious.

At this point, Lacan asks the following question: how can the wish to be free of guilt be what drives the dream, given that the wish is an extremely conscious one? It is after all Freud himself who confesses he wanted to be rid of blame, with the dream realizing this "wish." The unconscious wish that drives the dream must be a different wish.

Lacan wonders how Freud, who took the unconscious so seriously, could have settled for this interpretation. He therefore concludes that if the dream did indeed represent an unconscious wish, it couldn't have been this. The unconscious wish, here, was to be the founder of psychoanalysis.

In Lacan's analysis, the dream features the countertransference, which involves the therapist's feelings for the patient. Irma, Freud's patient, also happens to be a close friend of his and his family. Since, at this point in time Freud had yet to elaborate both the notions of (the patient's) transference and (the analyst's) countertransference, when Irma neither accepted his interpretation nor recovered, he simply resorted to considering her a "bad patient". In the dream she appears as someone who isn't quite right, something about her is "off." In the evening leading up to the dream, Freud had a conversation with his friend Otto, who later also appeared in the dream. Otto suggested that Irma's therapy had not really been completed and that there was more work to be done. This was what prompted the dream.

Lacan believes that the syringe in the dream introduces an element of coercion; it represents the wish to "inject" a solution into the problem – possibly by force – and thus to skirt the need for the patient to confirm the analyst's interpretation or subjectivize it. Lacan here identifies the psychoanalyst's desire as the desire to heal, as represented by Freud's colleague Otto who urges him to go on treating Irma. Since Freud has not yet considered the need to respect resistance, Lacan is led to define the psychoanalyst's desire exactly the other way around: the desire to release the patient from her expectations of the analyst as the Other.

The Real and Irma, and Freud's Desire to Encounter the Real

In Irma's open mouth, Freud observes something terrifying, an inner organ, with strange elements attached to it, something no one has seen before. The object is shapeless and uncanny. Lacan is surprised Freud doesn't wake from his dream at this sight, in horror of the Real. He wonders: what's so powerful about Freud's desire, what keeps him spellbound in face of this terrifying encounter with the Real? Another manifestation of the Real in the dream is through death and the fear of death, in the shape of Irma's illness, as well as being encoded in the name of the medicine Trimethylamine – the three Mathildas. In Freud's life there were three women called Mathilda, each of whom he unconsciously associated with the fear of death: his daughter, Mathilda, whose had suffered from a throat issue; a patient named Mathilda, who Freud feared he had prescribed wrong, harmful medicine, and another patient who went by that name, whom he had treated for anxieties, and who had died – though for unrelated reasons.

The developmental effort to cover up the Real by means of the Imaginary occurs in the mirror stage. Experiencing her or himself as fragmented and inundated by drives, the child identifies with their mirror image, which enables them to consider themselves one and whole. Freud the dreamer performs a similar move when he confronts true horror in the shape of Irma's symptoms, death, the shapeless organ in her throat – when he confronts all this by means of the Imaginary. In the dream, the Imaginary is represented through the other physicians, his colleagues, who appear as his parallels or doubles. Serving as his mirror image, they allow him to identify with the narcissistic role of the omniscient physician. This is how they "block" the Real's intrusion into the dream. The Imaginary protects against the horror of the Real.

According to Lacan, when the Real shows itself the dreamer usually opts to wake up. He is impressed by Freud who neither wakes up nor recoils. In doing so, Freud shows himself willing to face the "sphinx": incest, knowledge of infantile sexuality, and the unconscious; Oedipal desires and perverse urges – in short, the death drive itself. Freud was ready to recognize all this in relation to himself, to begin with. In this he anticipated his contemporaries.

Lacan only came after Freud boldly showed the way. Freud's courage, unlike Lacan's, wasn't about flying in the face of everyone else, but involved exposing himself and saying the truth, at the risk of being proven guilty. This is also why he is such a good writer. Lacan argued that key to Freud's choice to do analytical work was his determination to face the Real. The demand he addresses to Irma in the dream reflects this choice: he asks her to open up in analysis and confront her repressed drives. For Lacan, this exactly is the unconscious wish or desire the dream enfolds; the desire to face the Real.

Irma's Dream and the Creation Myth of Psychoanalysis, and Freud as Prometheus

In *The Interpretation of Dreams*, Freud mentions a patient who challenged his belief that dreams are about wish fulfilment:

> The dream showed that I was wrong. *Thus it was her wish that I might be wrong, and her dream showed that wish fulfilled.*
>
> (Freud 1900; emphasis added Y.I)

It is a well-documented clinical phenomenon that patients dream "for" their psychoanalyst, presenting material for interpretation. The unconscious produces subject matter for the session. Freud assumed patients were motivated to have a dream whose meaning would be "Freud was wrong" – hoping to communicate with and challenge him. This is the wish fulfilment in this particular dream.

A similar development, in Lacan's view, happens in Freud's dream about Irma. He points out that Freud's wish is to dream a dream whose meaning will be the founding act of psychoanalysis. As in the case of the woman whose suffering in her dream testifies to another wish, situated outside the dream, in her actual relations with Freud, the meaning of the wish in Freud's own dream, too, is located outside the context of the dream, in the very act of interpretation, writing and publication of dream interpretation.

Within the confines of the dream, Freud wanted his innocence to be proven in regard to an accident whose nature was physical, not mental. Outside the dream, however, in his interpretation, he blames himself for not having treated his patient well enough and for shirking responsibility through the "pretext" that the problem is a physical rather than a mental one. Lacan argues that Freud actually wanted to present himself as guilty and trying to evade responsibility. The desire this guilt represents is the desire to bring psychoanalysis into the world. Freud's admission of guilt in fact suggests: "If I am seen to evade guilt, that means there is something there to take responsibility for" – in other words, if it is possible that I am to blame for not treating Irma's unconscious adequately, that implies the unconscious indeed exists, and that there is a therapeutic method for its maladies, and this method is no other than psychoanalysis! The fact of Freud's guilt implies that it is not psychoanalysis, which is to blame for failing to cure, but the practitioner, who has not been using it properly. While Freud's guilt, on the narrative level of the dream, is about medical negligence, on the structural level it is a common, inherent part of any creation myth. In creation myths, guilt appears upon the arrival of something new – an event which, by the logic of exchange to which all language is subject, must have come at the cost of something else. Much like every child is "guilty" by virtue of their very birth, for giving their parents the trouble of raising them, in myths, the invention or discovery of something new – like the discovery of fire, art, or technological knowledge – is presented as somehow transgressive, a crime, a theft from the gods. Prometheus was severely punished for stealing fire from the gods and giving humans the knowledge that forms the basis of many crafts and technologies.

In the creation myths Lévi-Strauss collected from across the Americas, guilt is always accompanied by punishment for the appropriation or divulging of knowledge, often capital punishment. In the myth about the jaguar's wife, she is "sacrificed" in return for the knowledge of how to roast meat. Similarly, the mythology around Pythagoras, the philosopher, holds that when he discovered the famous "Law of Pythagoras," he sacrificed 100 bulls to placate the gods for the transgression against the gods. The same principle is at work in the Biblical myth of eating from the Tree of Knowledge. Knowledge is the province of the gods, not of humans. In crossing the boundary, humans change from being animals to being humans – something that brings them a little closer to the divine.

Like a Prometheus of psychoanalysis, Freud, by discovering the unconscious and inventing the talking cure, sacrifices himself. He does this by exposing his insufficiency as a healer. A punishment much less radical than the one suffered by Prometheus, yet Freud was fully aware of paying the price. He doesn't present himself as some shady charlatan, but as a good doctor who isn't scrupulous enough in applying a proven method.

There is another side to Freud's guilt, and this is that the knowledge he "stole from the gods" may be put to use for purposes he cannot control. This question reminds of the one as to whether the scientists who discovered nuclear energy should be held responsible for the untold suffering nuclear arms made possible. Freud expressed this type of sentiment in his conversation with Jung, on board the ship that took them across the ocean to America: "They don't realize that we are bringing them the plague" (Jones 1953). Freud was aware he was in possession of something explosive which could fall into the wrong hands. The infected syringe, in the dream, bears out the danger that knowledge also holds, and the fact that it cannot be controlled. Freud carries guilt for exposing humanity's instinctual, visceral qualities. It is exactly by situating himself as guilty for discovering the unconscious and establishing psychoanalysis, that Freud contrives to persuade us that there is such a thing as psychoanalytic knowledge, and a talking cure. Lacan's words, put into Freud's mouth, at the end of Chapter 2 – (Lacan 1988) capture this well. By subverting the hegemony of enlightenment rationalism, Freud comes in for further blame. The upshot was that he defined psychoanalysis as a type of resistance aimed at limiting the damage done by civilization (Freud 1930).

If Freud is guilty of stealing from the gods, this goes to prove that the knowledge involved is revelatory. If, by exposing the drive-infected syringe, he has transgressed against the censor and civilization, this tells us that there is both an unconscious and repression. And if he can be faulted for misapplying the method, that's proof there is, indeed, a method and that psychoanalysis works!

A Structural, Lévi-Straussian Interpretation of Freud's Dream

Had we presented Lévi-Strauss with Freud's dream, he may well have shown us how, since both rely on the structural laws of language, the same rules that obtain for the interpretation of myth are valid for dreams too. It's no coincidence that Australian natives call the mythic dimension of their culture *dream time*.

While Lévi-Strauss did not refer to the dream about Irma, Kuper and Stone (1982) published a structural analysis of it à la Lévi-Strauss. They pointed at the conflict between the biological and the psychic in the interpretation of Irma's afflictions and considered it a major focus of Freud's attention.

Read side-by-side parallels emerge between the dream about Irma as psychoanalysis' myth of creation and the creation myths Lévi-Strauss collected from all over the world. In both, representations of the transition from nature to culture are central, with the appearance of a Third constituting the dominant spectacle in this shift.

Creation as Triad and the Borromean Knot

Throughout his writings, Lévi-Strauss argued that all creation myths share a triangular structure. Things come into being as a result of conflict between two elements, requiring the emergence of a third by way of a solution. Differently put, things enter the world because the world needs them. Myths involving humans' discovery of new knowledge or technologies are in fact about the shift from nature to culture, and this shift is made possible by the Third.

Lacan regards the myth of Oedipus as another metaphor of this transition, describing human development in terms of the passage from being closely tied to the mother to becoming directed toward the father. Here it is the mother who represents nature, with the father, in the role of the Third separating between mother and infant, representing culture. The conflictual dichotomy, in Freud's dream, takes the shape of the question whether Irma's ailment is biological or psychological in nature: body or mind? Nature appears in the form of her physical complaints, and culture through her psychological ones. And as is common in myth, here too, in the myth that appears in the guise of Freud's dream, the aim is to resolve a clash between opposing principles. But how is this to be achieved? How do we reconcile body and mind, the biological and the psychological, Real and Symbolic? The solution is to maintain them both simultaneously, adding the Third to resolve the opposition.

In the Lacanian perspective, reality is a myth, composed of three dimensions or registers – the Real, Imaginary, and Symbolic – which are tied together into a Borromean knot. If we remove one element, the other two also come apart. It's like what happens when we saw off one leg of a tripod. The interrelations between the three are the key phenomenon.

Lévi-Strauss argued that in the basic structure of myth the Third enters as the solution to a conflict between two: the world therefore only exists in a formation of three. When one is missing, there is no world. Here we can see how Lévi-Strauss's thinking possibly influenced Lacan.

We might then ask ourselves, who represents the Third in Freud's dream about Irma? What is it that reconciles body and mind, Real and Symbolic? But before probing this question, let us first consider the role of the Third as cultural agent in myth.

The Third as a Cultural Agent – A Case from Papua New-Guinea

In Papuan myth, a boy-child who had sexual intercourse with his mother clings to her when she has to leave on her daily business. When he reaches the age at which he must leave his mother's home to live alone in the jungle in order to prove his masculinity, he must wear a "bride," a penis-sheath made out of palm leaves by women from an exogamous tribe – potential brides, legal candidates for marriage. But it is the mother who collects the raw material for the sheath, thereby signaling she is ready to let him go. It's as though tribal tradition and culture tell the mother: you're having a hard time separating from this boy, seeing him turn into a man. Therefore, you must participate in the process of separation with your own two hands.

In another version of this myth, the boy declines to leave his mother. He sticks close to her as she goes on her women's business and prevents her from picking the palm fronds from which she is supposed to make the penis sheath that announces his transition to manhood. The myth punishes those who resist maturation and separation from their mother; the boy is changed into a bird. Then, the bird defecates on the father's shoulder, and in due time, a tree takes root in this spot. To rid himself of the tree, the father creates water that divides bird from tree.

Often, myths will manifest interrelated systems that might reflect one another. In the above Papua-New Guinean creation myth, which actually recounts the origin of water, the son who is reluctant to leave his mother and transforms into a bird represents the kingdom of heaven. The tree that grows from the father's shoulder stands for the kingdom of earth – which always serves as a representation of the mother. And the water, in the role of the third element in this structure, divides between heaven and earth. Thus, this myth generates two parallel triangles: one relates to natural forces – water, earth, heaven – and the other to the family – father, mother, son. Water/the father are in the position of the Third, the function that mediates and separates between earth and heaven, and between mother and child. This myth functions as a creation myth for the origin of water.

In its typical layered mode, the myth articulates that the familial role division is part of a cosmic order, very much in the way that Freud situated the Oedipus as part of a universal law. This, in a nutshell, is what he did when Freud told Little Hans that he knew that Hans would feel his father as a rival and that he would love his mother, long before Hans was born because Freud knew that's how people are. Claiming that the law of the family is no different than the metaphysical principles of the cosmos is tantamount to saying: this is how it is, there is no other way!

The Scenes of Myth and of Psychoanalysis: Body, Family, and Couplehood

It is typical of myth to include correspondences between domains – the world of animals, the cosmos, the vegetable world and the human body. Lacan identifies a similar phenomenon in psychoanalysis, with the following three scenes mutually representing each other: the mother/child relationship, the couple's relations, and the manner in which parts of the body relate to the whole of it.

"The body" here denotes not just the biological organism, but also the body's surface as a sheet onto which structural relations with the other are inscribed. The parallel nature of these scenes enables crossovers; we can read what occurs in one scene as finding expression in another. So, for instance, a child's wish to detach itself from the mother can, in another domain, take the shape of giving up on a physical object; in the domain of couplehood it may manifest as an expulsive flare-up, and in the domain of the body as anal release.

Shifts between these different systems can occur when the unconscious cuts the dynamic from its original site to attach it to a representation from another. Physical constipation therefore may tell us about a child's unwillingness to detach from his mother. Lacan attempted to formulate an abstract structure describing the relations between child and mother, and between body part and the whole body. This pattern shows how different domains are parallel, and how elements take the same role, like father and water, which both serve as separating entities. For this purpose, Lacan borrowed the "golden ratio" from the field of geometry. The original ratio divides an object into two parts, such that the ratio of the whole to the longer part is equal to the ratio of the longer part to the shorter part (1:1.618).

The ratio is "golden" because it is considered harmonious, as borne out, for instance, in ancient Greek aesthetics. A modern version of the ratio is an A4 sheet. According to Lacan, this proportion in human relations renders the "precise distance" – neither too close nor too remote – between mother and child. This distance includes a tolerable degree of frustration – something that translates into other domains, and it is a sine qua non for entering language and culture.

The golden ratio's harmony is not merely predicated on the dangers of excessive intimacy or the inability to tolerate frustration: it equally implies the risk of premature separation. This suggests another version of the myth of the creation of water, where the husband, on discovering that his wife and son have had intercourse, strangles her and is subsequently punished. Here, the lesson is: Do not separate too early. The golden ratio, therefore, is not just the appropriate relationship from a mathematical perspective but is relevant to different domains, including nature and architecture, as well as the appropriate mental distance between mother and child, between body and body-part, and between couple and individual.

Freud's Solution: Sexuality as Third between Body and Mind

Let's go back to Freud's dream. We already mentioned a question the dream gives rise to: are Irma's complaints physical or psychological? Are they symptoms of hysteria, or is the issue an organic one? When we confront the mythic conflict between nature versus culture, the question arises of a possible Third who bridges between the Real and the Symbolic, between the biological and the psychological.

During the period when Freud had his dream about Irma, he was studying sexuality as an explanation for anxiety. In this context he coined the term *actual anxiety*, i.e., the outcome of an actual absence of sexual release. Physical frustration, he argued, transforms into psychic anxiety. Freud, therefore, situated sexuality between body and mind. Hysteria, too, the phenomenon from which he started his research, gives physical expression to a mental conflict. He defined sexual urge or impulse as straddling the boundary between body and mind.

Lacan's Solution: Language as Third

In the dream, the ostensibly physical diagnosis turns out to conceal a psychic one. A Lacanian interpretation of the moment when Freud takes a look into Irma's throat would be that Freud observes a "globus hystericus," or, loosely translated, that Irma has a "lump in her throat" – i.e., a psychic phenomenon. The dysentery also mentioned in the dream, about which it is said it will release toxins, parallels the catharsis of the talking cure, or as another of Freud's patients called it "chimney sweeping," the removal of toxic words through the mouth. The infected syringe – soiled, perhaps, by repressed urges – becomes a "solution" in the physical sense, a fluid into which some material has been mixed and solved, as well as a "solution" in the abstract sense of a fix. For Lacan, therefore, the Third tying together body and mind is not sexuality but language, the signifier itself. The appearance in the dream of the word *trimethylamine* indicates the solution is to be found in the signifier – in its very occurrence rather than in its meaning.

Meaning as Square-Shaped: Binaries Linking Domains – Retentive/Expulsive and Upper/Lower

At this point, let's revert to Kuper and Stone's structural analysis and to the analysis of Freud's dream about Irma. The tribal world view includes relations between various scenes and domains. We have witnessed this in the case of the Third appearing in creation myths, whether it is in the form of water in the natural domain, or in the role of the father separating, like water, child from mother – in the sphere of the family. A Lévi-Straussian analysis of the dream about Irma highlights universal mythemes, especially ones Lévi-Strauss collected in South America. What they have in common is the use of two binaries: upper versus lower, and the retentively closed versus the expulsively open. Whether the myth is dealing with the human body, forest animals, or cosmology, makes no difference. Similarly, it does not matter, in the dream, whether the events occurring in Irma's body map out a physiological, psychic, or theoretical constellation.

The mythic binaries of upper/lower, and expulsive/retentive are the codes by means of which myths or dreams narrate the transition from nature to culture. In the case of Irma this transition takes the form of a shift from the physical health of the body to the mental health associated with the symbolic domain of culture, i.e., the province of psychoanalysis. The upper element of the binary, in the case of Irma, is the mouth – whether open or closed; expulsive or retentive. The lower element is the anus, again in both states – open/expulsive or closed/retentive.

The formula of meaning is as follows: "The opposition between the upper parts' openness and closedness is like that between the lower parts' openness and closedness." This analogy enables us to point at a parallel with the process of healing: opening and release of symbolic toxins in the upper parts resembles the opening and release of physical toxins in the lower.

For native people too, the lower spheres are tied to nature, and the higher to culture, and they too use the open/closed binary. The distinction between nature and culture is reflected in the difference between earth and heaven, between lower and upper – in all domains and discourses.

One myth of the Takana tribe Lévi-Strauss studied tells the story of a sloth and a howler monkey who feature as each other's opposite and appear jointly to form one concept. As mentioned in the first chapter, in his earlier work Lévi-Strauss showed that concepts consist of binary opposites. In the local culture they denote the extremes of a spectrum, much like modern mathematicians use the symbols zero and one. The sloth is known for eating so little it doesn't defecate. In Freudian terms, this makes it anal-retentive. But the howler monkey, on the other hand, screams non-stop, and is clearly oral-expulsive. The myth introduces an opposition between expulsive and retentive, but not less centrally, one between the lower parts of the sloth and the upper parts of the howler monkey – the two extremes of the digestive tract. The original myth runs as follows: if the sloth goes against the myth and drops its excrement from high up in the tree – as the howler monkey is wont to do – then a meteor shower will come down on the world and destroy it.

Like dreams, myths too are not limited to the description of the event regarding the individual's or the animal's body. The high/low opposition is equally valid in the domain of cosmology, with meteors high up in the sky and showering down, and animals and cosmos are linked, as are plants and human bodies. In the category of "upper" are the mouth, the treetop, and the meteorites. The tree roots are linked to the anus and they both come under the "lower." Since the different representations of the same quality are interconnected, when a representation belonging to the "upper category" in a certain metaphor is altered this will affect a metaphorical representation belonging to that same category in another domain.

The upper/lower dichotomy in Freud's dream about Irma inheres in the feelings she reports in the upper part of her body, around her mouth, with which, of course, she speaks, as opposed to what she experiences in the lower part of her body, which are sensations associated with the animal aspect. When she opens her mouth, a growth is revealed that possibly bears similarities to parts of the lower body, so that upper and lower become superimposed.

In terms of structural analysis, there is nothing surprising about the appearance of the same topics of retentiveness and expulsiveness, upper and lower in both native myth and Freud's dream. This quaternary can be mapped onto Irma's body and ailments, much like it appears in tribal cosmologies.

Retentive and Expulsive Drives in Myths of Smoking, Laughter and Speech

Let's return to the native myths articulated through the binary tensions typical of the transition from nature to culture. A series of myths show the difference between expulsive expression or retentive withholding. Unlike its manifestation in the dream about Irma, where culture takes the shape of expulsive speech, in native myth, as in the illustration below, culture is represented by the restraint or suppression it demands.

In the Amazonian myth of the Kariri tribe, a fisherman slicing open the belly of a fish, discovers that it holds tobacco. At night he rolls cigarettes with this tobacco, but he smokes them alone, choosing not to share them with his friends. Smelling the smoke, his friends approach asking if they may join. When they smoke, however, instead of breathing the smoke out, they take it in. Both the fisherman's meanness, in refusing to share his cigarettes, and the friends' inhaling of the smoke render oral retentiveness.

At a later stage in the myth, the grandfather's spirit appears as a vampire bat (in other versions of the myth, it is an owl), who warns, if you don't exhale the smoke, you will be punished, for the tobacco is his. But the friends do not obey, and they are punished and turned into piranhas. Stinginess here acts to block the proper cosmic flow.

If we read this myth with reference to the three kingdoms (heaven, earth, water), and the Borromean knot tying them together, we see that tobacco derives from the earth, passes into water through the fish, while the smoke should rise up into heavens, the grandfather's seat. But when the smoke is inhaled rather than let out again, the Borromean knot is undone. Whether we are dealing with smoke, time, or any other object, the refusal to share interrupts the structure of exchange underlying language, kinship relations, as well as myth. Those who refuse lose their humanity and revert to the vegetal domain.

The myth about smoking has clinical significance because it refers to breathing. On the personal level the correlates are anxiety-related breathing dysfunctions, like breath retention, hyperventilation, or apnea. Close attention to the signifiers the patient uses when describing their breathing issues may reveal a story about the drive, whether expulsive or retentive, and the associated tensions, also manifest in eating disorders and other organic syndromes of boundary regulation.

Laughter in the Myth of the Origins of Animals, in the Myth about the Origins of Speech, and Freudian "Laughs"

The myth about smoking illustrates that to enter the domain of language we must give up on the object and share it. Another myth, this time from the Inuits, tells how long ago, there were only humans (Lévi-Strauss 1968). The monster-creator caught hold of some humans and tickled them. Those who managed to hold their laughter remained humans, but those who didn't and broke out into laughter morphed into an animal. Self-control, here, defines the human, and its absence signals the animal.

In a parallel version of this myth, a creature, half-howler monkey, half-human, has sexual intercourse with her son. Their offspring are the howler monkeys. And in yet another myth, humans, after using psychedelic substances, break out into uncontrollable laughter. Uncontrolled laughter, like incest, is transgressive behavior and therefore associated with the animal and vegetal world.

The North American Sioux tribe recounts how, after making humankind from the soil, the creator wanted to give humans speech. He ordered the humans to line up, introducing a small wolf whose role it was to make them laugh by attempting to catch hold of its own tail. Because this failed to do the job, the creator brought along a red frog that had a funny way of moving about. Only on his third attempt did the creator succeed in making them laugh and start to speak. Here, unlike in the earlier case involving tickling, laughter is already associated with communication, it is a kind of proto-language, situated in the symbolic dimension where human and animal are distinct. The configuration of the human line-up contrasts with the closed circuit formed by the wolf catching its tail and constitutes the principle of the chain of signification; the functions are fixed and can be variously filled, like in a sentence. Here we have the beginnings of the structure of language, from which culture, in its turn, can emerge.

Freud distinguished the kind of laughter that is expulsive and regressive, from laughter that requires the presence of a Third, that is tied up with the symbolic order, with culture. In *Wit and its Relation to the Unconscious* (1905) he compares the laughter evoked by slapstick, which requires two individuals – the one who falls and the one who laughs at the one who falls. For this it would be enough to watch the slapstick humor of the wolf chasing its tail without sharing the laughter with another human being. An example of the type of humor that is witty and requires the presence of another human being is the example of the frog who amused people in the Sioux myth: the fun poked at the frog is witty because it implies the joint assumption "Look at that funny frog!" while drawing a distinction between us-humans and the animal. A third, the object of laughter is required for cultural amusement to occur. Lacan quotes a witticism from Freud, the joke about the "famillionaire." Hirsch, who works as a bathhouse attendant, proudly boasts that Rothschild, a client, treated him "famillionairly" – blending together the two existing words, *family* and *millionaire*, to form a nonsense word. This is a witticism based on a slip of the tongue revealing the speaker's unconscious wish to be part of the family of millionaires. Here the joke is based on a Freudian slip of the tongue whose meaning is immediately obvious, and it operates on two levels: while it exposes the wish, it also allows us to laugh. Unlike the laughter produced by tickling, here a chorus is needed, or the recorded laughter used in sitcoms serving not only to cue the audience. The audience, in this situation, crucially needs (an) other(s) to laugh with, to turn the occasion into a cultural event. This type of laughter is distinctly cultural and in the symbolic domain.

It was Freud's choice to address the dream of Irma's injection as the founding event in the discovery of the unconscious, of psychoanalysis and the installment of the analyst. Like all myths of creation, here too, there is the phase of pre-cultural Real, taking the form in the dream of the strange findings in Irma's throat. The dream uses signifiers related to the body to demonstrate the building blocks of the structure of language. The open/close binary of the upper end of the digestive track is like the open/close binary of the end of the digestive track.

The Lévi-Straussian analysis of Amazonian myths shows us not only the underlying Freudian thematic of erogenous zones, but conversely too, how Freudian thought itself reproduces the mythical structure of all human thought.

References

Freud, S. (1900). *The interpretation of dreams.* Hogarth Press.

Freud, S. (1905). *Wit and its relation to the unconscious* (J. Strachey, Trans.). Hogarth Press.

Freud, S. (1930). Civilization and its discontents. In J. Strachey (Ed. & Trans.), *The standard edition of the complete psychological works of Sigmund Freud* (Vol. 21, pp. 57–146). Hogarth Press.

Jones, E. (1953). *The life and work of Sigmund Freud: Vol 2 Years of Maturity 1901–1919.* Basic Books

Kuper, A., & Stone, A. (1982). The dream of Irma's injection: A structural analysis. *The American Journal of Psychiatry*, 139(10), 1225–1234.

Lacan, J. (1988). *The seminar of Jacques Lacan, Book II: The ego in Freud's theory and in the technique of psychoanalysis (1954–1955).* (J.-A. Miller, Ed.; S. Tomaselli, Trans.). Cambridge University Press.

Lévi-Strauss, C. (1968). The Origin of Table Manners (Vol. 1 of *Mythologiques*). Harper & Row.

Lévi-Strauss, C. (1988). *The jealous potter.* University of Chicago Press.

Chapter 8

The Myth of Oedipus

Yehuda Israely

The myth of Oedipus has crucially accompanied the unfolding of western cultural history. Its role became even more prominent in the twentieth century, when Freud used it in his interpretation of the workings of the human psyche. For him Oedipus is the main myth expressing humans' unconscious drives, the two foremost of which are sexuality and aggression, as they initially make themselves known in the most elementary domain, namely, that of the family: sexual desire experienced for the one parent, and competition with the other. This chapter takes a deeper look into this myth, and considers differences and similarities between Freud's, Lévi-Strauss's, and Lacan's perspectives on it.

Freud's Oedipus – The Myth of the Rise of the Family

The structural approach holds that people take set roles in the family structure, as a result of which the relations among individuals within the nuclear family are, to an extent, dictated by these inherent patterns. Incest is a structurally anomalous relationship. It leads to a situation in which roles multiply; if the son has sex with his mother and she conceives a child, then this child will be both brother and son, while the mother is both mother and spouse. This breaks the first condition of structuralism where each individual occupies only one role.

In psychoanalytic theory, Oedipus is the family's "myth of origins". The prohibition on incest institutes and determines the structure of the family, including the nature of the relations among its members, in a way that ensures the family's continuation and replication in future generations. Prior to the importance Freud attributes to it in individual psychic development, and – in Lacan's model – to the paradigmatic absence at the origin of subjecthood – the myth of Oedipus represents an anthropological-evolutionary logic. It is about the catastrophe that ensues when the basic law of humanity is broken. Similar to native myths tying together human actions with natural events, in the myth of Oedipus the sin of incest brings a drought upon the city. It gives an account of the fatal injury to the order of life, to the very possibility of

DOI: 10.4324/9781003773764-9

engaging in productive, fertile living, that follows such a fundamental offense against the law. Freud, who discovered infantile sexuality in his clinic, and identified the attraction and competition between children and their parents, used the Oedipal myth to describe the unconscious conflicts attending these phenomena.

For Freud, over and beyond the family, the myth of Oedipus served as a template for the whole of human culture. The foundation of authority relies on the familial precedent of the Oedipal father. Freud believed that a person's coping with, and overcoming of, the Oedipus complex, is part of their development. Here she or he learns to let go of their regressive yearning for their mother, to accept the law of the father, which will eventually become the law of culture.

In the work of Lacan, Oedipus is a metaphor for the signifier's involvement in actual life, the Real. Surrendering *jouissance* is a condition for the subject's existence as a speaking subject, and hence: as part of humanity. And conversely, when language-based existence becomes compromised, as it does in the case of psychosis or trauma, this belonging to humanity, too, is fundamentally eroded. In the Oedipal process, the individual, who eventually identifies with the parent with whom they first competed, learns to reproduce the structure of the family and in adult life this will enable them to occupy the same role. This is true for boys as well as girls and also holds for the "reverse Oedipus," where competition is with the parent of the other sex.

For Freud the myth of Oedipus was the fundamental myth – or at least the main one. Both Lévi-Strauss and Lacan took different approaches. While in his earlier work, Lacan closely followed Freud, in his late seminars he took a different path in relation to the Oedipus complex and the role of the Oedipal myth. Lévi-Strauss, by contrast, and unlike Freud, chose to focus on the taboo on sexuality between siblings rather than on that between parents and their offspring. For Lévi-Strauss, therefore, the myth of Oedipus is not canonical as it is for Freud. At a later stage in this chapter, we will dwell some more on Lévi-Strauss's interpretation of the myth of Oedipus.

Lacan's Oedipus – The Father too is a Human Being

Freud argued that as she or he becomes more clearly situated in the internalized as well as the actual family, and with their assumption of the law of the father, the child enters the culture's symbolic domain. As the child receives their position in the family, it is received within the culture, or in other words, by becoming included in the ranks of the family we learn to live in myths. Lacan disagreed with Freud about the concreteness of the family processes required for the individual's entry in the Symbolic order. In Lacan's view Oedipus was a metaphor in which the mother represented nature, with the father taking the place of culture. This move away from Freud's concrete family relations to Lacan's relation of subject to language is notable in

Lacan's seminar "Joyce the Symptom" (1975–1976), in which he discusses James Joyce who mocked psychoanalytic readings of literary works on account of their reductionism. By explaining the creative impulse, he argued, psychoanalysis diminishes its importance, treating literature as a dream in need of interpretation. Joyce frequently used word and language play and thought that Freudian interpretations of slips of the tongue were missing the point. Lacan agreed with much of Joyce's criticism. He saw Freud as an advocate of the father figure, while Joyce presented an example of someone who could manage without one. He considered Joyce's psychic structure to have been psychotic, which means he did not undergo the Oedipal process as Freud described it, while maintaining the personal myths that enabled him nevertheless to take part in a symbolic reality.

The mythic structure Joyce created unfolded along the time axis. Loosely paraphrased, Joyce said something like this: "My father was a weak drunk – not a figure with whom I can identify. I'm looking for someone to identify with. Who will it be? I'll identify with a future figure of my own making! I will write world famous literature which will be read and studied into the next century. That's me – this admired future author! While it was Joyce's decision to have a future name, the interpretation that this was a solution to paternal absence is Lacan's (1975–1976). Joyce did become a world-famous author whose novels are still being read and taught. But it is important to remember that the proof of the power of the personal myth he wrote, rather than in his real-life success, lies in the fact that he lived and worked, assuming this future identity in which he invested so much energy. Joyce inserted death where the Oedipal father should have been. While acknowledging his own future death, he was going to have a "name" beyond it.

Lacan interprets Freud's interpretation of the Oedipus myth. He believes that Freud's Oedipal wish to kill the father is rooted in the assumption: "If I don't kill my father, he will forever remain the supreme master." Underlying this, says Lacan, is a belief in the father's immortality, in other words: He will not die a natural death. He must be killed if he is to die; to come down he must be made to fall, and to be removed from his throne, he must be treated without respect. Lacan questions all this. Will the father live and dominate us forever if we don't rise up against him? Isn't the father just another human being? Lacan reads the position of the father in exactly the opposite way; he reminds us that the myth of Oedipus concludes with the king losing his sight, something that underscores his mere, deficient humanity. According to Lacan, Freud refuses to see the father's humanity, which is reflected in the fact that he, too, is castrated. Unable to acknowledge the father's lack, he has to imagine him as non-castrated. This Lacan associates with Freud's biography, namely with the fact that he was ashamed of his father, which led him to seek, unconsciously, to elevate him.

Lacan believes that Freud's interpretation of the myth of Oedipus is informed by his own wish. In his "Interpretation of Dreams" (1900 p. 430),

Freud recounts a dream linked to the myth, leaving it unclear whether the dream was told to him by a patient or was his own. Many scholars have understood it to be Freud's dream. In the dream, the dead father appears as alive, conversing with him as usual, but (and this was the remarkable thing) he had nevertheless died, though he did not know it. The dreamer feels sad from the thought of having to tell his father that he is actually dead. On the death of his father, Freud wrote that a father's death is the most significant event in a man's life.

Lacan (Freud 1985) quotes from a letter Freud wrote to Fliess in which he says he himself identifies with the myth of Oedipus, and that he assumes these are universal feelings. But Lacan disagrees with what he considers a universalization. While the child's wish to be close to the mother is universal, he isn't sure whether the love–hatred conflict with the father, which Freud makes very prominent, is really shared by all humans.

The "Anti-Oedipus" and Humans' Engagements with Language

Lacan's work, up to a point, can be seen to reflect an approach we might call the "anti-Oedipus." This is the context for his reference to Malinowski's anthropological study of the sexual behaviors of Trobriand natives, who don't observe a traditional Oedipal-familial structure of the kind typical in the west, and who have sexual intercourse without any kinship-related constraints. He also quotes Durkheim who argued that the mother-child-father triangle is not universal (Lacan 1963–1964). Some cultures are marked by female dominance, some by male dominance, with husbands only occasionally visiting the family, and so on. The variety of family structures is so broad we cannot claim the Oedipus pattern is ubiquitous and the myth universal. Michel Foucault took this further when he argued that the Oedipal narrative was driven by a capitalist ideology that seeks to position the, preferably male, master in charge. This chauvinist-capitalist approach echoes the ancient master–slave model, which also includes father–child relations in the patriarchal Oedipal family.

Even so Lacan did not think the Oedipus was irrelevant. He wished to read it differently. For him the Oedipus myth is a familial metaphor for the human subject's relations with language. On this view, the mother in the Oedipal scene represents nature, the Real, the pre-Symbolic, with the father standing for language, law, and culture. Here the Oedipal transition from mother to father spells abandoning the Real for the sake of the Symbolic, a concession of bodily pleasure for the sake of social participation.

Lacan, the postmodernist, used the main Oedipal components to serve as an analogy for the relations between word and thing. The child's separation from the mother for the sake of its bond with the father is a metaphor for the movement from thing to word. In this way, Lacan poured Lévi-Straussian meaning into the Oedipus myth, as for Lévi-Strauss this exactly is myth's fundamental function, to render how the Symbolic detaches itself from the Real. Often, in native myth, this idea takes the shape of disengagement between animal and human. This is one reason for the fact that the totem constitutes the primal father in animal shape. We evolved from the animals, but the taboo on the totem signals we are no longer there.

Oedipus as Inspiration for the Healing Use of Myth

Over and beyond his discussion of the particular myth, Lacan also approached the Oedipus as an illustration of how myth – any myth – can be put to constructive, reparative use. Lacan believed that if psychoanalysts can show how they conceptualize what happens with the patient in terms of the Borromean knot linking Real, Imaginary, and Symbolic, this enables them to do what Freud achieved by means of the Oedipus: to conceptualize the unfolding of a patient's life by using myth. Whether psychoanalysts can produce a conceptualization of myths depends on their professional expertise and theoretical capacity. In this, Lacan follows Freud, but rather than using the ready-made myth, this insight works to stimulate mythic conceptualization within the clinic.

Conceptualizations of this kind may take the shape of interpretation of a symptom, its translation into myth, or the creation of a new myth. The new myth is a kind of "supplement" to which we introduce the patient in the absence of an existing myth – and Lacan calls this supplement the *sinthome*. Sometimes we may want to analyze a patient's story not merely to find out of what it consists, but to add something to that story with the aim to compensate for a failure in one of the registers – for instance, with a psychotic patient, in the Symbolic. We then introduce a type of fourth, prosthetic register, that serves as a patch, a supplement that enables functioning when the symbolic function is weak. A *sinthome* can for instance be a religion, ideology, or any belief adopted allowing Real, Imaginary and Symbolic elements to join into a coherent account of reality.

The Transition from Oedipus to Exogamy as a Dimensional Leap

The Oedipal exchange principle is a closed circuit: father loves mother, mother loves child, and child loves father. The mother must reconcile herself to a thankless role. The more successfully she raises her child to be autonomous, the more decisively the latter will turn to the father, instead of cleaving to her. Girls, to identify as women, will have to make a further transition by returning to the mother. The mother must somehow be compensated by the father for the child's departure. What we have here is a triangular, cyclic movement. This is equally true for non-heterosexual families, including single-parent or single-sex families because the respective roles in the triangle can be taken by others who are not members of the nuclear family. But the increasing number of family configurations testifies to the limits of Oedipal explanations.

The shift of Freud's Oedipus to Lévi-Strauss's exogamy takes us from three to four: the exogamous exchange principle opens up the closed, nuclear family. Exchange relations grow increasingly complex and what started as the exchange of sisters evolves into the unification of kingdoms through marriage.

The fourth position, in exogamy, is allotted to the maternal uncle. But in more abstract terms we may say the fourth member of the exogamous structure is death. Always, structure aims beyond the individual life. It is through the uncle that the nuclear family is tied to the community, an identification that seeks to solve the problem of death, a sort of immortality transcending individual identity.

Freud does not distinguish between the Symbolic and the Imaginary father as does Lacan. When the patient talks about castration, the limit of pleasure, it is the Imaginary father he has in mind. In this the Imaginary father resembles the archaic father who permits himself the pleasure he prevents from his offspring. This is the source of the master's discourse, the authoritarian-patriarchal mode, as well as the son's illusion that were it not for the restrictions imposed by the father, his access to pleasure would be unlimited. The Symbolic father, by contrast, is a method rather than an individual. While a person who identifies with the Imaginary father will say: "This is not allowed because I say so!" one who identifies with the Symbolic father will say: "This is not allowed because it's against the law and I too must obey it!" Here it is: the fourth element, the law, which represents the limit to which we are all subject, and which, in fact, is another representation of death. Death erases all hierarchies. Whether it's a Mercedes or a Fiat, both will have to wait in a traffic jam. In the face of death, the father has no edge over the son.

Even though the Freudian myth of Oedipus seems to address the survival of the individual suffering castration anxiety, rather than the future existence of the community, death, still, is arguably the hidden fourth element of the Oedipal structure, whose rule-based nature, similar to that of exogamy, ensures its own reduplication and the generational continuity of family and clan.

Still, at least on the face of it, the Oedipal structure leaves out the fourth element. By depositing authority over the weak son with the powerful father, it enshrines a neglect or disregard of the death that will eventually be faced by both. "The demand of the other" is the Lacanian term for the subject's fantasy regarding authority's claim on her or him, enabling them not to have to question their own desire. This question emerges when, in the face of death, it takes this shape (Lacan 1959–1960).

Freud's and Lacan's Actual Fathers – Between Authority and Radicality

Freud's simultaneously special and denied relationship to the paternal is manifest in his introduction to the Hebrew translation of "Totem and Taboo" (Freud 1913):

Authority, intelligibility, the conscious, the one – all united in the figure of the Oedipal father – are on the side of the "master's discourse." The psychoanalytic discourse, by contrast, is marked by the absence of external authority, the unconscious is structured as a network of signifiers, plurality, nonsense, while the Oedipal father stands exposed in his lack, himself castrated too, like any other subject. Freud, in formulating his Oedipal theory, was not the only one who was affected by his personal experience – so was Lacan. Their respective approaches to the figure of the father were linked to their personal desires in relation to it. Freud's Jewish monotheistic roots are tied to his tendency toward a single father figure – driving him to look for a single truth in his clinical studies. Lacan, who had received a Catholic education at a Jesuit-run school, moved away from the one to the trinity of the Real, Imaginary, and Symbolic registers making up the subject. For Lacan truth is less the outcome of investigation than a construction, and nor is it as monolithic as the Oedipal father.

Freud's myths of the father who tries to evade castration are Oedipus, "Totem and Taboo," and *Moses and Monotheism*. They testify to Freud's consideration of the father, to his desire for this type of non-castrated father. So, if "Totem and Taboo," for instance, illustrates his dream-father, it reveals a father invulnerable to castration; the father castrates all other men, and is eternalized after his death.

The myth of the father-exempted-from-castration in the case of Lacan belongs in a logic that produces meaning that sustains desire. In his Seminar "Encore" (1972–1973) Lacan discusses "Totem and Taboo"'s father who takes limitless pleasure in terms of the comparison between phallic and feminine *jouissance*. Phallic pleasure is grounded in lack because one can desire only when one lacks something, while female pleasure derives from desire itself rather than from its momentary satisfaction. While unlimited pleasure is expulsive, pleasure whose expulsiveness is bounded involves a retentive pleasure, pleasure in desire itself. If the subject is to define him or herself as lacking, they make use of the following, unconscious, logic: "As a rule, all humans are damaged and lacking, and since I am human, I too am damaged and lacking." But since every rule is externally defined by an exception, a male figure who is exempt from castration must be invented and defined as follows: "There is one person for whom the condition of castration does not obtain." This definition of the exception determines – from the outside as it were – the group of those who are subject to desire. This is the super-man, object of envy of all men who do not wish to know he has no existence outside their imagination.

Lacan subdivides the Oedipal father figure in terms of the three registers: the Real father is the person who contributed his sperm and the Imaginary father is the persona of the authoritative, didactic figure whose pleasure is unbounded. Unlike this Imaginary figure who asserts: "I am the law," the Symbolic father is ushering the child into the law and subjects himself to it as well. The Symbolic father represents the system.

His novel interpretation of the Oedipus also reverberated in Lacan's interactions with the psychoanalytic institutes. It was only after being banned from the International Psychoanalytic Association on account of these novel ideas and practices, that Lacan came to think of the Association as authoritarian, something which he then associated with Freud's authoritarian ethos. This change allowed Lacan to idealize Freud less, be more connected to his negative transference toward him, and recognize his limitations. This gave him the courage to distance himself from Freud and the Psychoanalytic Association.

Lacan's way of setting psychoanalysis free of Freud's patriarchal desire was by treating the father as a metaphor, a phenomenon in language. He was seeking to replace paternal chauvinism with a paternal metaphor. Unlike Freud, the Jew who wished to join the non-Jewish elites, Lacan was born privileged, son to an established Catholic, bourgeois family. Lacan's family context included a tyrannical grandfather who was in charge of the family's vinegar business and treated Lacan's weak father with cruelty. This combination of being from a socially higher-class background and having no master directly above him led Lacan to be more subversive, critical and radical than Freud. It enabled him to be more disrespectful against the culture of his origins.

Instead of his father, who had failed to do so in the face of his grandfather, Lacan took it upon himself to criticize the master (Roudinesco 1990). It was to be his way with most representatives of authority, including Freud and the International Psychoanalytic Association. His wish for an accessible, strong father, free from a grandfather's humiliations, he described in an encyclopedia entry on "family complexes." Here he presented his support for the "nuclear patriarchal family" because he believed it was on the basis of intimacy with an "accessible patriarch" that "creative subversiveness" flourished.

It is against this background, too, that Lacan identified with his hero Spinoza, who also rejected the master–father discourse. Rather than a natural, pantheistic divinity, Spinoza's God is the Jewish *hashem* – literally: *the name*, and one of God's several designations in Judaism. This divinity, however, is associated with neither personal providence nor personal claims and hence it lacks both authority and mastery. Having renounced the idea of a demanding orthodox Jewish God, Spinoza was able to situate desire with the subject rather than with the Great Other. By removing God's claim, Spinoza defined desire as the human essence. In so doing he set himself apart from rabbinical Judaism which puts desire on the side of God, while the apex of human achievement is to be an obedient servant. Where Freud situated the sublime father, Lacan placed castration. Castration, the outcome of us being speaking beings, includes us all, the father too. Lacan hereby takes back the tragedy to its original, fated state. This uncouples the father's death from murderous Oedipal desires. Fathers simply die, just like anybody else, and they lose their phallic grandeur much before that. If Freud had visited Lacan to undergo psychoanalysis, the latter would have had to help him pass the transition he called: "from impotence to impossibility." In other words, from a sense of being castrated in the encounter with the phallic father, to a sense of commonality based on the fact that we are all speaking human beings.

One of the most significant moments in a therapy arrives when a patient can say: "It's not up to me. I can do nothing about it. It's in the hands of fate and I have no guilt to bear." Taken a few steps further, this idea leads to the acceptance of death. After analysis, one can die with a quiet heart. In the transition from impotence to impossibility, or from failure to helplessness, failure must be left behind. We must give up on failure because failure invokes the fantasy of full satisfaction. This is also one way of redefining when analysis can be terminated. For Lacan, this is the moment when there is certainty about the inevitability of lack.

More on Oedipus and Lacan – On Knowledge and Truth

One interpretation Lacan elicits from the story of Oedipus concerns how little human individuals are aware of the story in which they live and which determines their fate. This reflects the discrepancy between knowledge as a system of relations between signifiers tied up in the signifying chains that produce the subject, on the one hand, and truth, which is the mode of subjective existence in speech. This interpretation of the myth of Oedipus is that the myth concerns castration as the divide between knowledge and truth. Truth, for Lacan, is a person's experience, whereas knowledge is constituted by the signifying system in which they dwell and which, unbeknownst to them, controls their fate.

The language in which the subject lives consists of interlinked signifiers which produce meaning. The most fundamental type of relationship between signifiers is that between first and second signifier. Lévi-Strauss showed that signifiers can represent elements from various domains – whether myth or social discourse. Both knowledge and truth are modes of relating between subject and signifiers. The first signifier is the one that represents the subject, enabling participation in symbolic-social discourse. It supports the subject's being and symbolic existence. It allows her or him to exist as one who expresses themselves and hence maintains the subject in her or his truth. The second signifier defines who the subject is, thereby reducing their being. Here we observe the signifier's coercive aspect. The second signifier includes all signifiers that follow it: the symbolic destiny of the subject. While the first signifier enables the speaker's active side, the second signifier, controlled by the Symbolic order, is tied to the passive position of the spoken. About this Freud said that psychoanalysis seeks to reduce the damage done by civilization, or in Lacan's words: to separate the first signifier from the second.

To revert to the myth of Oedipus – in Lacan's view Oedipus himself is subject to the knowledge, under which he lives. Oedipus neither knows whom he kills, nor with whom he sleeps, and in this sense, he is unaware in what story he features. Because Oedipus is willing to know, he convinces Tiresias to reveal the reasons for the plague. When Lacan admires Freud for being willing to know he puts him on one line with Oedipus, the hero. Unlike his colleagues, Freud is willing to know about Oedipal drives, infantile sexuality, and about repression – which is the refusal to know.

We can think of the blinding of Oedipus as a symptom, i.e., a statement through an act. The symptom says: "I was blind about the knowledge with which I lived." His revenge on having lost his vision is by turning a blind eye. The sphinx presents Oedipus with its riddle: "What walks on four legs in the morning, on two at midday, and on two in the evening?" The answer is human beings: initially they crawl on all fours; they walk on both legs in adulthood and support themselves with a stick in old age. The sphinx, who asks the riddle, is a hybrid creature, half human, much like the jaguar-woman in the myth about the origins of the cooking fire, whose role it is to die to abolish the overlap between animal and human. When Oedipus delivers the correct answer, he kills the sphinx, thereby removing the creature that straddles the animal and human. With the death of the sphinx, the human is inaugurated, and with it, there is knowledge and guilt. But even though Oedipus knew that the correct answer to the riddle was "humans," he didn't recognize that this included himself. King Oedipus, who vanquishes the sphinx, is the master whose *jouissance* knows no limit: whoever stands in his way is doomed to die. In this he resembles the archaic father of "Totem and Taboo." He fails to observe the gap between knowledge and truth. He does not distinguish the narrative of which he is a part.

Sophocles' trilogy – *Oedipus the King, Oedipus at Colonus*, and *Antigone* – describes how both the plot as well as Oedipus' knowledge develop. In *Oedipus the King* Oedipus still walks on two legs: what he does not know is that his fantasy of the almighty king is doomed and that he will become crippled, and in need of a stick. This is what happens to him in the second tragedy. The name Oedipus itself, which literally means "swollen foot," suggests that castration in the form of crippling inheres in his name from the outset, long before he becomes king. *Oedipus the King* concludes with failure. He fails to avoid the Oedipal sin, as if the matter was in his control. The second play ends in helplessness. Here Oedipus acknowledges his mistakes, but he does not go beyond feeling helpless and denying his guilt. Oedipus disengages from his image. He divests himself of his titles, his honors, his public role, saying, as it were: "I have managed to free myself from what was imposed on me." To some extent this releases him, as said, from his (self-) image, the signifiers that have determined his fate.

Flashes of this kind occur during psychoanalytic therapy: when suddenly a person is capable of taking an external perspective on the narrative into which they were born. Then the statement is: I agree to being the hero of this story, and as a result I gain more freedom to choose something in it, including a role to which I attach myself.

Lévi-Strauss on Oedipus: Myth about the Origin of Humankind

In his interpretation of Oedipus, Lévi-Strauss did not limit himself to the well-known Greek version. He also included ancient Mesopotamian myths in which he identified four mythemes which can be found back – in slightly varying versions – in the myth of Oedipus:

Dangerous intimacy between blood relatives, as in incest.
Extreme alienation between relatives, like in blood feuds.
Monsters emerging from the ground.
Heroes with names referring to humans originating from the soil.

If Freud understood the Oedipus myth to be an account of the emergence of the family, Lévi-Strauss took it to have a broader scope, namely, the emergence of humans. He asks whether humans originate in the flesh, sexuality, and family, or from the inanimate earth.

The first two mythemes (incest and blood feud) represent the basic instincts of sex and violence. From these drives – through their curbing and organization – human culture emerges. In this sense humankind is the result of reproduction, family conflict, and the drives. The other two mythemes (monsters, connection with names), by contrast, point to another reading: here human beings are not the mere product of their family, they have origins in nature itself.

The monsters coming out of the ground are part human, part animal, symbolizing the close ties between humans and the animal world. So, when the hero of a myth slays a monster, it is, in fact, the connection with the animal that is severed, stating: No longer am I part of that wild natural world. Thus, as we've seen in the Amazonian myth, the hybrid creature that's half jaguar and half human is killed to represent the moment when the human individual, by cultural necessity, sets her or himself apart from animals.

Once this cut from the animal world has been achieved, the fourth mytheme, referring to humans' new connection to the earth, appears. This connection has now become human rather than animal, something which is signaled through the heroes' *names*. Oedipus's name, for instance, implies a limp, something that tethers him to the ground and to matter. A human being, made of dust, and no longer an animal. The story of the origin of humankind thus refers to three sources:

From flesh and blood – the outcome of sexual and violent relations between blood relations
From the animate world – which the human individual must leave behind
From the soil – the stuff of creation, from which humans are made and to which they will return

The link between human and soil features not only in ancient Greek myth but in many other archaic traditions. In the Jewish genesis, for instance, the first human is made out of dust. And Sumerian tradition has it that the gods Anki and Ninhursag forged the first human out of clay – which is the material from which the rest of the world, too, was made. This is because humans must be part of the world: rather than just inhabitants, they must be made from the very same material.

This relationship between humans and the world surrounding them – they are a product of that world and not external to it – forms the basis of animistic beliefs which see human beings and the universe as connected entities.

An even more ancient myth of creation found in many cultures, from eastern Europe to Australia, is about a waterbird who dived deep into the ocean and brought up a chunk of earth from which the entire world unfolded (Eliade 1963). This myth may well have accompanied mankind from the onset of its wanderings out of Africa, tens of thousands of years ago.

Even contemporary science finds a place in this portrayal of things: modern astrophysics shows that the components of the human body derive from the stars, from the furnaces of ancient supernovas.

We started this chapter with the question of how the myth of Oedipus deals with humans evolving from both a mother and the earth. Lévi-Strauss approaches this by claiming that the Oedipus myth gives no precedence to either side of humans' origins, biological or cosmic, by including both. While the myth formulates this tension, it solves it through a narrative: The human being emerges from *both* its mother *and* the soil of the world. Birth from the mother renders the familial, biological, and instinctual, the place where life originates but which holds many threats (incest, violence). Birth from the earth, by contrast, implies a wider range of belongings: to the world, nature, the entire universe. In this manner, Lévi-Strauss's reading of the myth of Oedipus bridges between the personal – family ties – and the universal – belonging to the world.

Cadmus, Oedipus, and Antigone

For each myth to which Lévi-Strauss's studies led him, he identified and outlined its mythemes. The mytheme of extreme family closeness, distant and even aggressive family relations, and encountering monsters that spring from the earth, are repeated in the myths of the Oedipus lineage.

The first myth in the sequence talks about Cadmus, the archaic father of the dynasty that founded Oedipus's city of Thebes. Here the mytheme of family relations is reflected in Cadmus's search for his abducted sister Europa. The mytheme representing monsters erupting from the earth takes the shape of Cadmus battling against a dragon who rises from the ground. The Spartoi – brothers who fought and killed each other – spring from the teeth of the monster which Cadmus planted in the ground, yielding the final, missing mytheme of blood relations.

The second myth Lévi-Strauss analyzed is the myth of Oedipus. The mytheme of excessive closeness in that narrative is represented by the incestuous relations with the mother; and distant, even aggressive relations with the father he did not know, while the monster emerging from the earth is the sphinx. As concerns the fourth mytheme – heroes named in relation to humans being created from the soil – all the heroes of this dynasty carry names that convey disability or injury associated with the leg: Cadmus's grandson, Laius, his son, and Oedipus, son of Laius. A limp signals someone who has only recently sprung from the earth – a universal, cross-cultural motif of the period.

Finally, Lévi-Strauss looked at the third of Sophocles' tragedies, *Antigone*, where he identified the aggression in the war between the brothers who kill each other and the extreme closeness in Antigone's resignation to being put to death in punishment for having buried her brother.

The mytheme that deals with humans originating from the soil and eventually returning to it, here takes the form of Antigone's acting under the obligation to bury her brother and thereby restore him to the earth even if she will have to sacrifice her own life to do so. Eventually she is locked up in a subterranean cave. The name Antigone, however, does not continue the motif of the crippled leg: *anti-* against; *gona-* offspring. Her name might indicate that Oedipus's dynasty ends in her generation.

And as for Antigone, similar to Oedipus being Freud's hero, Antigone can be said to have been Lacan's. She embodies the ideal of taking one's desire beyond the limit. Antigone is willing to die to maintain the honor of her family by burying her brother. By identifying with a principle, Antigone makes her life meaningful over and beyond mere survival. This is a mythic way of pointing beyond death. About this, Lacan says that what was created in the first death survives the second death (1992), or in other words, the signifier that replaced the subject, reducing its vitality, is the very thing by means of which the subject can conceptualize and immortalize itself.

Antigone-type thinking plays a role in the clinic: a patient ended up having to care for her old father even though he had made her suffer throughout her life. Her Antigone-like solution was to look after him for the sake of the value she attached to family life rather than directly for him. Antigone is willing to die and be buried in the belly of the earth so that the signifier "family" will persist after she is gone. As she identifies with this act, which reaches beyond death, she ties herself to eternal values. Had Antigone failed to bury, properly returning him to mother earth, had she not returned his soul to the tribe's collective bundle of souls, she would have transformed her own lived life, retroactively, into an existence outside of the signifier, lacking structure or community. This would have retroactively canceled her as a subject. Having to choose between organic and symbolic life, she preferred the latter dimension over the former.

Freud's, Lévi-Strauss's and Lacan's Shared Oedipus – Eternity

What is the common thread between these interpretations, Freud's, Lévi-Strauss's and Lacan's? How do we connect between Freud's notion of the family, instituted on the basis of the prohibition on incest; Lacan's version concerning the impossibility of bridging between the Real and the Symbolic, between truth and knowledge; and Lévi-Strauss's account of humans' emergence from either reproduction or the soil? Can we identify a shared motif?

In the first chapter, discussing Lévi-Strauss's methodology, I described how, when seeking to understand why twins were taboo in the Amazonas, he had to go all the way to Vancouver, Canada to find an answer. Twins are associated with hares, whose upper lip is split, while they themselves, too, are the result of splitting, this time inside the mother's womb. These narratives share the fact that when a symbol of perfection is required, splits are under taboo.

In the case of the myth of Oedipus, it may be a good idea to follow Lévi-Strauss's methodology by looking for other myths, somewhere on the "psychoanalytic continent," in our attempt to explain the common denominator between these variants. Unsurprisingly, the question that has always preoccupied humanity, appears in Freud's, Lévi-Strauss's, as well as Lacan's versions of the myth: it is the same question on which the archaic myth of Gilgamesh centers, too, namely that of eternal life.

Immortality for Freud is the outcome of the taboo that enables the generational reproduction of the family. It is no coincidence that Oedipus's children consumed themselves, bringing Oedipus's family line to an end. For Lacan, immortality is of the signifier which replaces the subject. Eternity or immortality, in the case of Antigone, is reflected in the act of identification with timeless family values. And as for Lévi-Strauss – it is the return to the earth, in the mythic context of emergence from the earth, that presents death as a return to the mother's lap, where one is shielded from the danger of death.

Let us now look at myths, both native and psychoanalytic, that support this thesis, showing Oedipus as a myth of immortality. For this purpose, we will consider the Amazonian myth about the sexual origins of death; and as regards psychoanalytic myths, we will discuss the archaic father in "Totem and Taboo" as well as the death drive in *Beyond the Pleasure Principle*. In the work of Lacan, we will engage with the principle of eternity through the myth of the Lamella.

Journey Between Myths of Eternity

Myth of the Erection and Death – The First Death Survives the Second

In Amazonian myth the first man created is perfect. His sexual organ is in a state of constant erection. The first woman teaches him how to relieve this erection by means of intercourse, undermining his perfection. God is angry and punishes the humans who are now mortal and must beget children (Lévi-Strauss 1969).

The message of this Amazonian myth, then, is that orgasmic sex issues in death. Those who continue to live a time-bound life, banned from eternity, are a new type of creature, the product of combined parental genes. Parents are bound to die, and soon enough, so are their offspring. If death is inevitable, the myth makes it more tolerable by introducing a deal in exchange for becoming mortal, humans get the pleasure of sex and another form of immortality through generational continuity.

Lacan's statement, "what was created in the first death survives the second death" holds the same meaning as the Amazonian myth. The first death is of the thing that the word replaces, as when the older child gives up on a sweet for the sake of a younger sibling and in exchange, as it were, is called "big girl" or "big boy." Here the "title" replaces the pleasure of having the sweet itself. The second death is that of the organism. Though this second death is the ultimate Real, the more a subject identifies with signifiers, persisting beyond their personal, organic death, the more of an effect of immortality they will achieve.

Lacan's Lamella – Unicellular Immortality

Death and sex came into the world together. Prior to the arrival of sexuality into the living world, creatures did not die a natural death. Unicellular organisms persist through infinite splitting. Lacan uses the *lamella*, an imaginary unicellular organism he invented, as a metaphor for the infinite nature of signification. Lacan's myth of the lamella complements the myth of Oedipus by associating immortality with not just the reproduction of the family structure but the very essence of language-based human life. It is identification with the signifier, via the metaphor of the undead unicellular organism, that offers the interface with infinitude.

In Freud's work the Symbolic order, of which the law is a major element, initially appeared in the form of the superego. The superego, for Lacan, however, is only one expression of the Symbolic. The signifier too serves as a basis for structure, which enables life-in-narrative. Because it is not animate and cannot, therefore, be killed, the signifier is immortal.

But, though the lamella holds out a kind of immortality, it represents a dangerous perfection because it negates the subject who is based on lack. The lamella is the object of our yearning for the thing whose loss has doomed us to sexuality and death. It is the threatened fulfilment of our regressive wishes, which is the stuff of nightmares. Like the "Nothing" in *The Neverending Story*, it spreads like a dark stain, relentlessly. And the lamella also represents the lost object, the *object little a*, which we will discuss regarding Little Hans's phobia.

Freud's "Totem and Taboo" – When the Archaic Father is Replaced by the Eternal Totem

In "Totem and Taboo" Freud presents the following myth about human history: a group of apes were living according to the law of the jungle. The alpha male was the father, all female apes fulfilled his pleasures, and the other males, his siblings, were in the clutches of envy. It was the discovery of organization that spelled the transition from ape to human. While the single male is too weak to topple the leader, when males bond together, they can confront him. And so, all the father's sons joined to kill him, and the strongest of his offspring inherited the leadership. In no time, however, the other brothers joined in struggle against the prevailing male and killed him. If, earlier, there was nothing to constrain the father's boundless desire, now there was nothing to curb the power of coalition. None of the brothers wanted to be the father's heir because it was obvious that this would mean their immediate death. Since humans are crueler than chimpanzees, there was no chance it would be limited to a ritual struggle. But humans are also more intelligent than apes, enabling the males to make a coalition that outdoes any single alpha male in strength. As a way of breaking through this murderous cycle, a myth was invented in which the clan's leader is presented as totemic symbol rather than as an ordinary mortal.

The emergence of the totem followed the same logic as the emergence of the third: to settle the conflict between the two – between the alpha male and the coalition of siblings. The myth of "Totem and Taboo" which Freud invented is a parable explaining the transition from nature to culture. It is the Freudian-mythic version of Lacan's principle whereby the signifier killed the thing and then replaced it. In the case of Lévi-Strauss, the alpha male is substituted by the totem signifier, which represents membership of the family or tribe. But unlike Freud, for whom the totem was the sculpture itself, the specific signifier, Lévi-Strauss regarded it as method or structure.

Since the totem is not a living thing, it cannot die or be killed by rivals to the crown. The totem is the crown, and it is immortal, even if the one who wears it keeps changing. To ensure the survival of the clan, a non-living leader, who cannot therefore die, is appointed, a leader who is not human and hence exempt from rivalry and envy.

In their correspondence between the two world wars, Freud answers Einstein's question about a solution to war, by repeating this idea as key to world peace: democracies must join together against dictatorships, like the siblings against the father. In this context, the United Nations is mentioned – who also initiated the correspondence (Burton 2002). The UN could be the totem representing the community of nations, replacing the father whose *jouissance* knows no limit. Instances nowadays of the totem include God, the church, the constitution, the presidency, but also charms, or mascots representing soccer teams. While the real leader is beyond human she or he is represented by the incumbent. The pope, for instance, is not merely the leader of the Catholic world; he is imbued with the power of St Peter.

Beyond the Pleasure Principle – The Death Drive and the Myth of the Inanimate Returning to Itself

In *Beyond the Pleasure Principle*, Freud discusses phenomena like shell shock and post traumatic disorder. Why would a person choose (even if unconsciously) to return in their dreams, night after night, to a burnt tank? He wondered whether the logic of this nightly replay of an impossible situation was an attempt to solve it. Maybe this time the surviving soldier will manage to save his injured comrades? Or could the over-excitement of the situation trigger some masochistic pleasure, a type of agitation ostensibly the inverse of the organism's tendency to homeostasis?

Lacan introduces clarity in his explanation of the nature of the symptom. Like other types of symptoms, the post-traumatic symptom consists of an envelope and a core. The envelope is symbolic – suggesting that repetition, for instance "the attempt to find a solution," is meaningful – while the Real nucleus of the symptom is included in this envelope. Here repetition is tantamount to *jouissance* – though this may not be consciously registered. But let's first address the question why the organism strives for equilibrium, homeostasis, reduced excitation? To answer this question, let's return to a myth Freud invented and which we already mentioned in Chapter 4: Life originates in the inanimate. The living cell consists of inanimate molecules. One variant of this myth is the dictum, in Genesis: "From dust you came and to dust you shall return." Freud adds the positive yearning of matter to return to dust. This suggests that the lifeless is not truly without life; what we have here is not the physicists' entropy where it is in the nature of matter to disintegrate. In Freud's myth, desire is projected onto matter which strives to return to a primitive state. And this animistic myth is, in fact, no other than the pleasure principle. This is one form the death drive takes: the myth of the living thing's yearning for stasis, absence of tension – a state of inanimateness. This relies on the animistic belief that lifeless dust is a type of living matter and hence the return to dust implies immortality.

Earlier mentioned hyperstimulation is the opposite of this will to stasis. In looking for suffering and tension, beyond the pleasure principle, masochism rejects the inanimate. Leading to ecstasy, however – itself a kind of annihilation – hyperstimulation, too, invokes the death drive. Putting together this myth with two other Freudian myths – Oedipus, and the archaic father – we can see that they share the point that humans' structural tendency to seek excessive pleasure – whether it takes the form of absolute serenity, according to the pleasure principle, or of absolute stimulation, as under the principle of beyond the pleasure principle – threatens the structure of the family with collapse.

Between the extremes of nirvana and total excitation, a certain degree of non-gratification gives room to desire, access to language and use of communication, family and community life, as well as a degree of tension involving a rejection of the inanimate-nirvana state. It is only in language that "nothing" can gain the status of "something" and thus transmute, lack can transform into desire, thereby avoiding nirvana, on the one hand, and ecstasy on the other. A dog, when hungry, suffers. His consciousness will be preoccupied with the absence of food. Human consciousness, unlike its canine cognate, operates by means of signifiers, and language can produce an ontologically opposite idea. Over and beyond *no-food* as dogs too experience it. Human language allows for this possibility: "I have what there isn't". The sentence "Once I had depression and now, I have desire" is only possible in human language. It is only in language that the absent can take the status of present. Presence and absence are both, and simultaneously, underwritten by language, which rejects ecstatic states of absolute absence as well as inanimate states of absolute presence.

Myth as Deal – What's the Price of Immortality Through the Signifier?

We can see that all these myths feature a deal. What do we give up in order to get what the myth promises us on the other side of our sacrifice? At what price do we acquire the signifier of immortality? According to the Freudian Oedipus, the child, in exchange for losing out to the father in the struggle for the mother, gains membership of the family, and eventually, through identification with the father, the ability to function, himself, as a father. He will be able to raise a family, with offspring of his own. In *Antigone* Sophocles makes very clear what price the eternal signifier involves, when Antigone willingly accepts her own, personal death for the sake of her brother's memory and the continued existence of the hallowed family.

In "Totem and Taboo"'s myth of the archaic father, the potential for unlimited *jouissance* is lost, but in its stead community solidarity appears. Forgoing tyranny and absolute pleasure yields brotherhood, law, constitution, and identification with a totem assumed to have qualities of immortality. Identification with a community holds out the everlasting. Juxtaposing the myths of the archaic father and of Oedipus results in the following idea: in constraining the son's *jouissance* the father produces desire; the principle of social organization that puts a limit to the father's *jouissance* issues in community. Language and culture replace bodily pleasure and the law of the jungle.

In *Beyond the Pleasure Principle*, language, instead of the serenity of the inanimate and the ecstasy of stimulation, makes possible the desirous existence of life that emerges.

What's the cost of identification with the Lamella, which releases us from the death imposed by sex, and holds out immortality through identification with the signifier? We pay in terms of *jouissance*. When the signifier replaces the thing, it becomes a part object – incomplete in terms of such *jouissance* as remains. The immortality of the pre-sexual, unicellular organism is replaced by the sexual, multi-cellular, human organism's word, language, speech, symbol. Immortality is lost with the arrival of sexuality and regained with the introduction of language. For animals, we might argue, death does not exist, because they have no consciousness of death. Immortality, for animals, is therefore redundant. While language makes death conscious, it also affords a myth of immortality. Much like in psychoanalysis, myth presents solutions in language to problems that arise in language.

References

Burton, H. (Ed.). (2002). *Why war? Einstein and Freud's little-known correspondence on violence, peace, and human nature.* Basic Books.

Eliade, M. (1963). *Myth and reality* (W. R. Trask, Trans.). Harper & Row.

Freud, S. (1985). *The complete letters of Sigmund Freud to Wilhelm Fliess, 1887–1904* (J. M. Masson, Trans.). Belknap Press of Harvard University Press.

Freud, S. (1900). The interpretation of dreams (A. A. Brill, Trans.). In J. Strachey (Ed. & Trans.), *The standard edition of the complete psychological works of Sigmund Freud* (Vol. 4 & 5). Hogarth Press.

Freud, S. (1913). Totem and taboo. In J. Strachey (Ed. & Trans.), *The standard edition of the complete psychological works of Sigmund Freud* (Vol. 13, pp. 1–162). Hogarth Press.

Freud, S. (1939). Moses and monotheism. In J. Strachey (Ed. & Trans.), *The standard edition of the complete psychological works of Sigmund Freud* (Vol. 23, pp. 1–137). Hogarth Press.

Lacan, J. (1959–1960). *Seminar VII: The ethics of psychoanalysis* (J.-A. Miller Ed., D. Porter, Trans.) W. W. Norton & Company, 1992.

Lacan, J. (1963–1964). *The four fundamental concepts of psychoanalysis* (J.-A. Miller Ed., A. Sheridan, Trans.). W. W. Norton & Company.

Lacan, J. (1972–1973). *Seminar XX: Encore* (J.-A. Miller Ed., B. Fink, Trans.). W. W. Norton & Company, 1998.

Lacan, J. (1975–1976). *Seminar XXIII: The Sinthome, or Joyce and the Sinthome* (J.-A. Miller Ed., A. R. Price, Trans.). W. W. Norton & Company.

Lacan, J. (1992). *The seminar of Jacques Lacan, Book VII: The ethics of psychoanalysis, 1959–1960* (D. Porter, Trans.). W. W. Norton.

Lévi-Strauss, C. (1969). *The raw and the cooked* (J. Weightman & D. Weightman, Trans.). Harper & Row.

Roudinesco, É. (1990). *Jacques Lacan & Co.: A history of psychoanalysis in France.* (J. Mehlman, Trans.). University of Chicago Press.

Sophocles (2002). *Oedipus the king* (R. Fagles, Trans.). Penguin Classics.

Chapter 9

Little Hans and Animism

Yehuda Israely

Little Hans was the youngest of Freud's patients. His father, an admiring student of Freud's, consulted him about his 5-year-old son who had developed a phobia of horses. Relying on a description of the father's conversations with his son, Freud advised how to approach the child's distress. This case description has served as a prototype for psychotherapy with children, but it also shows how human and cultural development – including little Hans's mental development – unfolds through phenomena we know from the domain of anthropology, like animism and totemism. Just like native myth, the myths Hans invents and around which his phobia organizes itself, are specific, addressing a taboo. And the very same myths, in the versions Hans forged as his father listened, were what eventually got rid of the phobia from which he was suffering.

In the myths Hans produced, the phallus appears in various roles. He is preoccupied by his "widdler" – his penis. He gives himself pleasure until his mother puts a stop to it. She puts the fear in him, threatening castration. Hans displaces his fear to a horse. The horse's widdler is more impressive than his own, and Hans fears the horse might bite him. Another thing that perturbs Hans is his discovery of sexual difference. Upset by the possibility that his mother doesn't have a penis he assumes it must be hidden somewhere between the folds of her flesh. One reason that Hans takes fright is that for him, the phallus signifies living beings. He wonders how it is possible that his mother lacks this thing. This is how Hans defines something as alive – even an inanimate object like a train carriage. As he watches a train carriage move by, he says – as if explaining to himself – that its phallus too is "invisible," it simply happens to be "hiding" right now.

How does animism operate? Why do children and natives take it for granted that everything around them is imbued with a soul? What, indeed, is a soul? And how do the soul and Hans's widdler stand to each other? How are body and soul connected?

DOI: 10.4324/9781003773764-10

Smoke Stands to Meat as Soul Stands to Body and as Signifier Stands to Thing

Amazonian natives recount how, at first, the spirits allowed men to hunt and eat raw meat only. Then humans discovered the secret of roasting meat over the open fire. Next, they acquired the skill of cooking meat in a basket filled with stones heated on the fire, and after that, when earthenware pottery fell out of the skies, they placed the pot directly over the flames to cook the meat. Now came the next stage of preserving meat by drying it, using salt, and finally the technique of smoking arrived. In Amazonian mythology body and soul are tied together as meat and smoke. When meat is smoked, the flesh itself vanishes, leaving smoke only. Meat is like the body and smoke like the soul which continues to exist after being removed from the perished body (Lévi-Strauss 1969). Given these pregnant meanings associated with smoking, the important cultural status of smoking becomes evident; it is an iteration of the smoking of meat. The practice comprises the whole sequence of culture emerging from nature, from raw meat down to the production of smoke in the absence of meat.

Smoke, in addition, resembles the signifier which "detaches itself" from the actual thing, gaining a life of its own in the domain of signifiers. In Chapter 2, we mentioned how Helen Keller experienced this when she described how, through her darkness of sound and vision, she first understood the nature of words; now each new object she touched and felt seemed to gain life as she gave it a name. Once she sensed herself surrounded by signifiers rather than just "things" she felt them stirring with vitality. She felt this about the signifier "water" with its direct sensory correlate, but no less with abstract concepts like "God" or "love," which are not tied to the "meat" of the actual. This is in the nature of the totem, which, though originating in the flesh-and-blood archaic father, is, like smoke or the soul, a signifier that has survived the death of the Real object.

So, we may observe a chain of meaning unfolding, based on analogy between pairs of opposites: as smoke arises from meat, the soul arises from the body, and in the same way, too, signifier arises from object. The latter – signifier arising from object – is a myth whose function it is to explain the signifier. This myth recounts how signifier, in earlier times, was attached to object in the same way as smoke is connected to smoked meat. Only later did it acquire a separate existence. The truth is that the signifier was at no stage attached to the object. It is the sign, for instance the onomatopoeic sound – the sound of the word *drip*, or the visual shape of an arrow – that began by being linked to an actual phenomenon and then became detached. The signifier, by contrast, doesn't derive its meaning from the thing itself but from other signifiers. Lacan illustrates this with the image of two doors: on one of these, it says "men" and on the other "women." These words obviously refer to the gender difference between people who are heading to the toilet, but they carry meaning only in so far as they serve in opposition to each other. Each door, therefore, only has meaning in so far as it functions in opposition to the other.

The myth about the separation between body and soul, like the separation between object and signifier, gives rise to the concept of the soul, both on the level of the subject and on that of the things surrounding us. For everything that has a signifier, there is "soul," namely eternal life, untethered to the physical body. As natives, and little Hans, see it, everything, all things, possess soul. And just like signifiers exist through mutual affirmation, the same goes for all that has a soul. The signifier exists in a web of signification, and similarly the soul exists in a network of reciprocal relations among souls. Just like there is a universe in parallel to the universe of things – namely the universe of signifiers – so there is a universe parallel to the revealed universe, namely the universe of souls or spirits. The souls of humans, jaguars, and rivers, as well as the souls of the dead, are all linked together in one grid. This is how animism places the subject in exchange relations with the world. The subject is represented to others by a signifier, and these others in turn are similarly represented by signifiers. Like brides in exogamy, or like gifts passed among Trobrianders, signifiers can be exchanged, and the same goes, therefore, for the things they stand for. In this they function like commodities on the market which, once they acquire value in a common coin, can be traded. If the other is a signified like me, and hence in possession of vitality like me, we can acknowledge each other as having desire and exist in an exchange structure with a common currency; hence we have the ability to satisfy each other's desires. If we have a common currency we are made out of the same material, like people who share a blood type and can donate blood to each other, or people who speak the same language can exchange meaning. Animistic myths attribute language and expression to the surrounding world and through the solidarity of language, humans experience themselves as bound together in exchange relations. Exchange relations are especially pertinent in human interactions with gods through sacrifice.

Arguably, in our exchange relations with a god we have something to offer her or him, while receiving, in return, an answer to our prayers. Hans animates the world by attributing a phallus like his own to all, including inanimate things. The phallus defines its owner as a participant in the exchange market whose members are those who desire. For Hans, the phallus constitutes the shared symbol subserving the categorization of all living things. This is what leads him to expect others – whether humans, animals, or carriages – to be animate like himself, in possession of the same signifier of vitality, namely the thing he knows to identify with desire.

Referring to Aristotle, Lacan (1964) understood this as follows: the soul is humans' yearning, desiring part because thought is naturally drawn to take care of what is lacking. Hans ascribes to all things – to the carriage no less than to the horse that pulls it – the phallus, signifier of life or subjectivity. The phallus makes it possible to identify the other (whether human, animal, or inanimate object) as an agent of craving. But why should the widdler be the signifier of the soul? Hans dreams he touches his widdler as he looks at his naked mother – a moment marking the emergence of the sex drive. He feels, and hence knows, that this is his private organ of longing. Since the world is replete with beings that yearn in language, Hans's analogy is simple: They too must have a "longing tool."

The Hypothesis of the Subject's Intentionality

The subject is identification as a function of intentionality. If the ego is "I am seen, therefore I am," the statement "I intend, therefore I am" yields the subject. Subjectivity emerges with hindsight, that is to say, once the world ascribes intentionality to someone: this is when the subject as an intentional creature comes into being.

> "Daddy, the lightning is broken."
> "Broken?"
> "Yes. There's no thunder."
> Noa is three years old, and her parents smile.
> "Daddy, the lightning is off," she repeats and they laugh again.

When she commented on the lightning, Noa didn't intend to make the adults laugh. She really thought that when lightning isn't followed by a thunder, something is wrong, like a toy without batteries: the two have to occur in tandem. When there was the nice bonus of her parents' laughter, she repeated the question, but this time with the intention to make them laugh again. Noa understood her parents' reaction to mean they thought she intended to make them laugh. This is how an initially absent intention comes into being. What she will remember, later, is that she meant to make them laugh, twice over. The moment Noa believed she had an intention, she acquired the function of intentionality, which is to say, subjectivity, which is to say, a soul. First, human beings become animate to themselves, i.e., experience intentionality in themselves, and subsequently they invest the rest of the world with a soul.

Freud, on Hans's request, drew a giraffe, and next Hans asked him to add a widdler. Freud responded by asking Hans to do it himself. This is a good illustration of psychoanalytic technique. By encouraging Hans to act, Freud pointed to his agency, his subjecthood. Freud confirmed phallic ownership as signifier of Hans's subjecthood. In other words: "It's up to you. You own the phallus, you add it. You're the one who from your desiring perspective bestow desire on your surroundings." Though Freud did not directly link this intervention to the cause of Hans's phobia, Lacan points out their connection. For Lacan Hans's phobia is about excessive intimacy with his mother, whom he experienced as devouring because his father failed to fulfil the role of ensuring distance between them, or, in the present context: offering his own phallus to the mother. The subject risks being devoured, while the suggestion to produce the phallus himself underlines that he is a subject who can make choices.

Horse Phobia as Myth Organizing Family Intimacy

> "[…] but does he know everything that is in God's head?"

This is what Hans asked his father about Freud (Freud 1909 p. 43).

He wasn't all that wrong. Since his father was an enthusiastic follower of Freud, the transference relations also transferred to Hans. In the introduction to the Hebrew translation of "Totem and Taboo" (1913), Freud stated how deeply rooted he felt in his Jewish identity and that he had no wish to relinquish it. When, long before Hans's therapy, his father, who was Jewish too, considered converting to Christianity, Freud convinced him not to let go of his Jewish identity. Since, at that time, about half of German Jews were choosing to convert, Freud must have had considerable influence over Hans's father.

For Hans, Freud was part of the family. It was Freud who gave him a rocking horse for his third birthday, a horse that might have played a role in Hans's subsequent phobia. If Freud overshadowed Hans's father, and weakened his role as an authority who could separate him from his mother, it's only fair for Freud to have used this authority to release Hans. These biographical details present us with a background against which, for Hans, Freud's status was something like a "master." When Freud told Hans that, based on his knowledge of what people are like, he knew even before Hans was born that he'd love his mother and compete with his father, he was in the position to convey something that normalized Hans's Oedipal feelings.

Children are exposed to myths that organize family relations, for instance through fairy tales like "Goldilocks and the Three Bears" or songs like "This Little Piggy." This is what Hans does with his phobic symptom: as the natives, in Freud's myth in "Totem and Taboo," substitute the primeval father with the totemic animal, so does Hans with the totemic figure of the horse. Freud takes the horse to symbolize Hans's father, while for Lacan it is a symbol for both mother and father. Hans regulates a proper distance from his parents by mythical means and through the metaphor of the horse. The totem replaces the parental figure to repress the knowledge that the actual conflictual relations are with the parent(s) themselves. The symptom releases the individual from the need to be conscious of their conflicted feelings for their parents but in doing so produces the side effect of dysfunction.

The Horse as Father – Identification with the Father as Buffer Between Child and Mother

Phobias, according to Lacan, are evidence of failure in the paternal metaphor, i.e. substitution: something goes wrong in the developmental process of replacing mother by father, which occurs when the Oedipus complex is resolved. Hans's mother does not have sexual intercourse with his father, and she does not shield her son from the sight of her naked body. Hans fails to substitute his mother with his father and therefore feels threatened by her excessive proximity.

Freud mentioned three types of identification: identification through a shared signifier; hysteric identification through a common desire, and identification through an object that belongs to someone. Hans identifies the horse with his father by reference to a visual signifier, namely, the black patch – in the form of his father's moustache, and the horse's blinkers – each carries. What causes Hans – even if unconsciously – to turn the horse into a threatening figure? Lacan's answer to this question is that Hans needs a buffer between himself and his mother, instead of his father who is not powerful enough, both in relation to his mother and to Hans. Native people use totems for similar purposes: the totem replaces the archaic father who is not immortal. He was killed by his enemies who refused to subject themselves to his authority when he set limits to their pleasure. The totem, unlike the father, does not live, and is therefore not mortal: it is stable like the law which stays valid even after the lawmaker dies. This is the boundary Hans longs for when, unconsciously, he gives the horse the power to draw boundaries, however terrifying.

The association between father and horse emerges in a slip of the tongue, when Hans says: "xx". The father interprets: "xx". By doing so the father means to communicate to Hans that he loves him and isn't angry or vengeful, even though Hans has aggressive impulses toward his father. Hans reacts by laughing, indicating relief. One is allowed to have clashing urges. This laughter confirms that Hans's father's interpretation was right. As a result, Hans goes on to act as though he was a horse himself: he identifies with the father's totem.

The Horse as Mother – the All-Erasing Threat of Perfection and the Role of the Phobic Figure

The subject imagines that if only he restored his lost object, he would feel whole and perfect. He doesn't realize that if that were to be the case, he would not be a subject and feel nothing. The subject is grounded in lack. The threat of regression to fusion with the mother equals the threat of perfection. The danger of perfection is that it erases the subject, as the latter is a function of intentionality – which cannot exist in the absence of desire (lack or need, in other words). The well-known custom of producing a flaw against the evil eye, like breaking a floor tile on moving into a new home, serves a number of purposes in native thinking. This marring of perfection seeks on the one hand, to avert malevolent envy, as well as, on the other, to serve as a sacrifice to the gods invoking their protection. Creating a fault has another meaning in the context of family relations where it gets in the way of incestuous fusion with the mother – one of the forms of perfection.

The boy in Amazonian myth who refuses to separate from his mother, accept her gift of the penis-cover, and participate in coming-of-age rituals, is punished (Lévi-Strauss 1969 p. 44). In Chapter 2, discussing the myth of the subject's creation, we described how the proto-subject orbits the object and how the empty-handed return constitutes the moment of the subject's emergence. In Chapter 8, dedicated to the myth of Oedipus, in the discussion of Lacan's *lamella*, we mentioned that identification with this unicellular organism, which is subject to neither sexual division nor death, promises a form of wholeness. This is exactly why it is dangerous to approach: the subject, after all, is grounded in lack. Phobia is one way of averting this danger of no-lack, of fusion with the incestuous object.

Freud relates to the horse in terms of the father only and never suggests it might also refer to the mother. For Lacan this is another expression of what he critically considers Freud's fixation on the father figure. He believed that Freud's intimidated respect of the father was so overbearing it prevented him from considering other interpretations. Lacan understood the horse to refer to both father and mother, and the fear of being bitten by the horse to express fear of being devoured by the mother. While the concrete background to the boy's fear is his mother's actually voiced threat of castration, it also involves the regressive urge to be seduced by the mother and have difference erased.

To install difference, the subject unconsciously situates the object, and the wholeness it promises, in space and makes sure to maintain physical distance by means of a shield, a screen that keeps them apart. While the screen itself is transparent, the phobic object – whether spider or horse – constitutes a kind of stain on this wall, warning the subject against coming too close to the mother behind the screen. When the fear of engulfment is formulated in terms of a spatial threat, this allows for a symptom whose anxiety can be resolved by taking physical distance from the phobic object.

Castration and Coping with Sexual Difference

Hans fears castration. He says to his mother: "I thought you had a waddler like the horse." Hans's theory concerning the animistic signifier does not fit with a reality in which his mother has no penis. Anxiety arises when a myth "doesn't work." It terrifies Hans that his mother might be imperfect. This would testify to a deeply flawed universe. If creatures without a penis exist, then he might lose his own; moreover, his mother has warned him that if he keeps playing with his widdler, "xx." Hans fears the loss of vitality that losing his widdler will bring about. Sexual difference is proof of lack. This is associated with lack in the subject, as well as in the Other with a capital O – two forms of lack the subject must engage. Hans and his mother were, mythically, whole. The encounter with sexual difference leaves both his mother and himself lacking.

To resolve his fears and contradictions, Hans concludes his mother must own a penis – it's just hiding between her legs and not always visible. He's also exposed to the anatomy of sexual difference through his little sister, a few months old baby, yet he insists that everyone possesses a widdler. Often, even after sexual difference is discovered, denial returns.

Serving to remove the threat of castration, this denial has some other functions as well. When young children play peek-a-boo, they delight in the object's disappearance and return. A similar pleasure in discovery, oblivion, and re-discovery can be observed in adults too when in the erotic act of undressing, they are aroused time and again, at the exposure of what is already known.

Little Hans's Recovery Through Myth

We said that the phobic symptom serves as a kind of myth that helps Hans put himself at a proper distance from his mother and father. But the price of this "xx" is compromised functioning. To let go of this symptom, Hans will have to produce alternative, more adaptive myths. The two following myths serve just that purpose. In the first, he will marry his mother while his father will marry his own mother, Hans's grandmother, that is. As a result, he will not be the only one to gain incestuous pleasure: his father, who surrendered his position, will do so too (Freud 1909 p. 97).

The myth does not have to come true. It suffices as an example of a hypothetic situation in which ownership of the mother doesn't cause Hans to have clashing feelings of hate and love for his father.

The second myth is about a plumber who will replace his widdler just as he does with the faucets: he will remove Hans's little widdler and substitute it with a big one. In the first part of the myth, the plumber's removal of the little widdler makes castration possible and for Hans to accept the separating father. The second part of the plumber's job, in which Hans receives the big phallus, enables identification with the father. Lacan draws attention to the fact that what eventually healed Hans and stopped his phobias, was neither the mere consciousness of his clashing Oedipal feelings, nor even Freud's universalizing the problem by saying he knew this would happen even before Hans was born. The symptom was eventually resolved when Hans himself formulated the myths. This is what we observe in our clinical work. Movement becomes possible when we introduce a myth supporting us in the face of the contradictions of existence, or when, interpreting a symptom, we identify such a myth. Now we might return to a case mentioned in Chapter 6, describing a patient who was unable to get over the loss of her dead husband. When she made a near-Freudian slip of the tongue, using the expression "my ex-husband," she suddenly referred to herself as a divorcee. The "divorcee" myth helped her to separate from her dead husband. The myth of divorce was more efficient in supporting her as she took leave from him than the myth of widowhood.

References

Freud, S. (1909). Analysis of a phobia in a five-year-old boy. In J. Strachey (Ed. & Trans.), *The standard edition of the complete psychological works of Sigmund Freud* (Vol. 10, pp. 1–149). Hogarth Press.

Freud, S. (1913). Totem and Taboo. In J. Strachey (Ed. & Trans.), *The standard edition of the complete psychological works of Sigmund Freud* (Vol. 13). Hogarth Press.

Lacan, J. (1964). *The four fundamental concepts of psycho-analysis* (A. Sheridan, Trans.). Hogarth Press.

Lévi-Strauss, C. (1969). *The raw and the cooked* (J. Weightman & D. Weightman, Trans.). Harper & Row.

Chapter 10

Repetition and Interruption

Yehuda Israely

What Was Lévi-Strauss Looking For?

As its name indicates, structural anthropology studies structures and patterns that repeat themselves in any given culture. In his research, Lévi-Strauss collected patterns, like motifs occurring across myths, or family structures that are reproduced from one generation to the next. Probing these patterns, he hoped to gain insights about human nature and culture. But aside from paying attention to structure and pattern, Lévi-Strauss did not lose sight of small variations in these myths' recurrent structures, and they drew his attention to the question of what happened when such changes occurred and repetition was broken? Acting like a "geneticist of culture" he began to identify "mutations" in iterations of formulas, equations of meaning, to probe whether it was possible to identify regularity in breaches of repetition, and whether such breaches could itself be captured under one, fixed structure. What he was really after was to find out the function of these discontinuities or interruptions in cultural myths.

In his research on post-trauma concerning his work with his patient Emma (Freud 1953), Freud, too, studied repetition and its disruption. Lévi-Strauss turned to this work for inspiration in his attempt to find order in human cultural phenomena. What was there for him to learn from Freud's thought about repetition and its disruption, its underlying mechanisms and regularities? Below we will take a look at the case of Emma, but before doing so, we might say that what Lévi-Strauss essentially took away from Freud was that it is only through the disruption of repetition that change and development, on both the individual as well as the cultural level, can take place.

The Case of Emma and Repetition in Trauma

Emma, a young woman who was being treated by Freud, told him how she remembered escaping a shop in a panic when she was a young girl. While she couldn't say why she had acted this way, she knew it was somehow connected

DOI: 10.4324/9781003773764-11

with the two young men who had laughed at her dress, when she entered the shop alone. She was twelve at the time, and her reaction had become generalized over time so that now in her early twenties she avoided entering any shop on her own. Recollecting that earlier event, Emma commented to Freud that one of the two salesmen was nice-looking.

The memory of her visit to the shop led Emma to remember another, earlier event, when she was eight, which happened in the very same shop. She remembered how the shop manager grabbed at her genitals through her clothes and smiled. She blamed herself for returning to the same shop in spite of what had happened there. Listening to what the young woman was telling him, Freud paid attention to the details she mentioned in linking the two recollected incidents. Emma's associations guided Freud to the common element: it was the laughter of the two shop assistants which took her – at age 12 – back to the shop owner's smile when she was eight. Another such element was her being alone. She had been alone in the shop during both incidents. "Alone" was one signifier in the triggering system. Freud assembled the signifiers featuring in the narrative about the 8-year-old and explained how they repeated themselves when she was 12, gaining traumatic meaning. The signifiers that were repeated between these two points in time were *shop, laughter, clothes, alone.*

Trauma, here, unfolded over two phases. First, when Emma was 8, there was the trauma-inducing event of the manager touching her genitals, but only when she was 12 did it register as traumatic. The threatening core during the first-stage trauma was being an erotic object to a stranger. Though eight-year-old Emma was unfamiliar with post-pubescent erotic excitement, she felt it in her body once she was 12, when she experienced shame and distress facing the two salesmen, yet a glimmer of sexual attraction too. Only then was she able to know what she had experienced when she was eight – knowledge she had repressed until the meeting with Freud.

As I explained in Chapter 3, which was dedicated to the emergence of meaning, something can only mean anything by comparing it to another thing. For Lévi-Strauss, to be precise, meaning emerges when four signifiers configure an analogy between two oppositions: the relation A to B is like that of C to D. The meaning of the word "cold" will be "indifferent" where the four elements constitute an analogy between the opposites: "warm stands to emotional as cold stands to indifferent."

As repetition, eventually, consists precisely of these four elements, its formula will include eight elements. The earlier mentioned quaternary formula, *the relation A to B is like that of C to D* repeats itself in, *the relation E to F is like that of G to H*. Lévi-Strauss called this octagonal structure the "canonical structure." Yet he pointed out that this repetition is interrupted with a certain regularity. At the eighth point, *point H*, something changes: a passive position gives way to an active one. I will expand on this presently. Let's first look at

Emma's story in terms of this formula including elements arranged into two quaternaries.

In 8-year-old Emma's experience she **sees** (A) the **smile** of the salesman (B), much like she **feels in her body** (C) the man's **perturbing attraction** (D). In this manner the smile came to mean perturbing sexual contact. At age 12, repetition occurs: Now Emma **observes** (E) the young men's **laughter** (F), similar to how she **feels in her body** (G) **how she is attracted** to one of them (H).

The first sentence in each of the two quaternaries obviously constitutes a full repetition: Emma observes the salesman's smile, and four years later she notes the two young men's laughter. But while we expect a simple repetition of perturbing attraction, now Emma actively experiences her own sexual urge, rather than being victim to that of another person.

This trauma unfolds across two points in time. When she was eight, at the time of her actual trauma, Emma may have had some understanding of something not being quite right in the interaction with the salesman, but she could not understand its meaning for him. The event registered as something the mind was, as yet, unable to decipher, and is tied up with the primary trauma of not-knowing. The next point in time occurred four years later, when Emma was 12, with the incident involving the two young salesmen, a scene that repeated some motifs of the first incident: laughter, clothes, alone, in the shop.

Now that she had experience of her own sexuality, she understood the nature of the other salesman's behavior, four years earlier, and that she had been the object of his sexual impulses. If we did not conceive of trauma as the subject's involvement in what happens to them, we could have settled on the explanation that the young men's laughter reminded her of that of the older salesman, earlier. This, however, would only offer a partial explanation of what Emma went through. It was her own arousal on realizing she liked the looks of the young shop assistant that led her to fill the event four years earlier, where she had been the object of someone's *jouissance*, with traumatic meaning. It was, accordingly, only then that she began experiencing the phobia of entering a shop alone. What appeared now, in fact, when Emma was 12, was a double repression: she repressed both her impulse, and the association between that consciousness and the victimizer's sexuality. Emma's phobia emerged to keep her away from the danger zone, even if she was unaware of its nature.

Something else, over and beyond understanding, with hindsight, what had happened when she was eight, occurred during the repetition of the scene at age 12. Emma, from being an object, became a subject. This change found expression in the shift from noun to verb. We might say that what was repressed as holding danger was not merely Emma's memory of being harassed, but also her encounter, age 12, with her own sexuality. Years later, when she was 20 and went to therapy with Freud, he drew her attention to these transitions. In their conversation Freud dwelled on his observation that her subjectivity emerged when she felt sexual attraction: this time she felt attracted rather than being the object of someone else's attraction. This introduction of subjectivity and agency triggered a change in Emma's repetition compulsion. Freud's interpretation had highlighted subjectivity.

Subjectivation, or the subject's recognition of their erotic investment, is therapeutically valuable in the encounter with trauma. The treatment of trauma involves emphasizing the subject, their urges and choices. Attention to the subject's responsibility for her or his own wishes and needs, frees them from the position of the choiceless object – which is the traumatized position. Turning to activity, if it is interpreted in a way that enables the subject to own their drive, resolves repetition compulsion.

We might think of her psychoanalysis as the third point in time in the story of Emma's trauma. The first event happened when she was 8; then when she was 12 that event became traumatic, was repressed, and now the phobia manifested itself; in her early twenties she remembered her experiences at age 8 and 12. As mentioned, she did not observe a connection between these events and her phobia of being alone in a shop. Becoming aware, in conversation with Freud, of her urges, and of the resulting removal of repression, made the phobia redundant, and the symptom vanished.

Another way of approaching this is as follows: it is the role of myth to organize reality in a manner supportive of psychic needs. The formula of repetition with a twist in the plot is only completed when Emma reaches her twenties, thanks to Freud's perceptive observation that she was attracted to one of the young shop workers. This is when myth finishes with its psychic work, with Emma shifting from the object position in the first quaternary, to the subject of the second quaternary.

The story of Yehiel Dinur – or Ka-Tzetnik, his pen name – illustrates the same idea (Dinur 1987): trauma is resolved by taking a subject position. For many years, Dinur, a Jewish man who survived the Nazi death camps, suffered from insomnia, until he turned to LSD-supported psychotherapy. During a drug-induced hallucination he saw himself in Nazi costume, and following this his insomnia disappeared. Much like Emma's trauma was a response to another person's drives, Dinur, too experienced trauma due to Nazis' sadistic drives. Healing came about following his identification as the subject of his own drive. Gaining awareness of his own drives resolved the component of his anxiety that rejected recognition of those drives.

To conclude, the most consistent, yet surprising, element in all structures of repetition is that, eventually, it issues in a change or departure in the narrative. There is a point at which repetition deviates from itself in a very characteristic way: at the eighth point, or H, the subject in their active aspect emerges and upends repetition. This can be formulated as follows: the first round of repetition ends with the establishment of the object in the context of the analogical quaternary. The second round of repetition, however, concludes with the object being substituted by a subject. It is in the absence of the object that the subject, in fact, appears.

The Canonical Formula – in Myth and in the Clinic

Emma's case and the insight concerning repetition it afforded Freud, inspired Lévi-Strauss when looking at the mechanics of repetition in myth – something he called the "canonical formula" (Lévi-Strauss 1988). In his research on repetition in native myth, Lévi-Strauss identified some more features of how repetition is broken in them – in addition to Freud's discovery of the transition from passive to active. Lévi-Strauss's canonical formula defines repetition by means of two transformations. The first of these is the already familiar one from passive noun, as it appears in the first quaternary, to active verb, in the repeated, second quaternary. In the case of Emma, as we saw, this involves her change from "attractive girl" to a "girl who feels attracted." The other transformation Lévi-Strauss identified is that what was negatively charged in the first quaternary, takes on a positive charge in the second, repetitive quaternary. In his *Mythologies* he frequently dealt with mythical pairs representing binary opposites to illustrate the equation of meaning based on opposition, and the mechanism of the canonical formula. One of his analyses compares between a myth dedicated to the origin of clay, and one about the origin of pottery making. Below we look at Lévi-Strauss's work on these two myths to deepen our understanding of how alongside structural repetition, disruption of that same repetition occurs. We will pay attention to the two "transformations" he pointed out in the structure of meaning.

The Myth About the Bad Bird and the Good "Birding"

The first myth derives from the Jivaro tribe in the Amazon (Lévi-Strauss 1988), and deals with the origins of sun, moon, the diurnal cycle, and the source of clay. The story harks back to ancient times when sun and moon were not sky dwellers, but two earthly men married to one woman whose name was Goat Sucker. This is the name of a bird distinguished by its wide beak – hence its name: goatsucker. While the woman loved the sun's heat, she did not like the moon's chill. Jealous of the sun, the moon covered it causing a first solar eclipse, and then he rose into the sky. Now the sun, too, ascended in pursuit after the moon, and ever since, the sun and moon race and chase after each other in the sky, but never coincide.

Using serpents and creepers to hold on to, Goat Sucker climbed into the skies, following the sun and the moon. As she did so, some soil from the earth stuck to her. Her getting involved in a romantic triangle in heaven was, in terms of the myth, considered a breach of taboo: the serpents and creepers tore, and Goat Sucker tumbled back to earth together with them. In this myth, the creepers and serpents function to link the worlds below and above.

So long as they achieve this connection, they lead to harmony and perfection. When the woman, along with the serpents and creepers, falls down, this perfection is undone, and now heaven and earth are separated. In her fall, bits of clay come down along with her – and this is the source of the clay we use for pottery, which the myth comes to explain.

The goatsucker is a bird the natives consider to be greedy, a stingy hoarder. Known for its envious nature, the goatsucker features in myths about betrayal, jealousy, and marital strife. In certain myths, the goatsucker is also associated with themes involving the dissection of body parts or decapitation, rendering the cosmic split between the birds of heaven and the serpents of the earth.

Lévi-Strauss found another myth which corresponded inversely with the above, goatsucker myth, namely the myth of the ovenbird. The equation of meaning based on an analogy between opposites serves as the basis of this pair of opposing myths. In the eyes of the natives, the goatsucker and the ovenbird are each other's opposite, just like black and white, or like zero and one in current thinking. The myth of the ovenbird also involves clay, but differently, it engages with how pottery entered the world, the activity whereby raw clay is shaped into nice pots that are useful for humans. Identifying the repetition between these two narratives, Lévi-Strauss also noted how they diverged.

As mentioned, the transition from the quaternary of meaning to that where repetition is undone consists of a shift from bad-object, to good-action. The myth serves to define the goatsucker as an evil object. The good action that appears in the myth of the ovenbird must be a declension of the word "bird" from noun to verb. Something like "birding" well.

The ovenbird is an emblem of good marriage: It owes its name to the fact that it is faithful, doesn't tend to envy, and carefully builds its nest out of clay, its domed shape reminiscent of an oven. In the myth of the ovenbird, creatures who are part animal and part human, and who are the forefathers of the natives, the Matako tribe, go to visit the fire giants. The giants' children were squatting down behind their parents, kindling the fire. The ovenbird observing this, broke out into loud laughter. The giants' children, offended, went to their parents to complain. Incensed, the giants responded by setting fire to the whole world. To protect themselves, the natives imitated the ovenbird: digging a pit whose walls they covered with clay, they hid in it through three nights and three days, going without food. In contrast with the goatsucker, who builds no nest, sows division, causes fights and is greedy, the ovenbird is a good partner in marriage, builds a proper nest out of clay, and harmonizes. Here we can observe myth shifting from positive to negative meaning. However, another transformation, too, can be seen to occur: The myth features the evil goatsucker as a noun, whereas the ovenbird appears in the shape of a verb. The act of "ovenbirding" equals building a nest out of clay. With the act of overbirding, pottery enters the world of humans who learn the skill from the bird. The shift between myths indicates a corresponding move from evil to good, from a greedy, destructive bird, to one associated with a harmonious home; it also signals the shift from passive to active in the verbal declension, as laid out in the canonical formula. The transition from passive to active can also be detected in the myth's subject: from clay, a natural raw material, to pottery, in a creative act whereby humans use nature in order to produce a useful product.

Lévi-Strauss's research has been key to identifying homo sapiens' system of symbolic operation regarding everything touching the domain of the mind and culture. His work also broadly confirms Freud's discoveries concerning the role of repetition in trauma and adds its own contribution to psychoanalysis in the form of structural listening, a concept Lacan borrowed from him.

The Subject's Drive as Response to the Demand of the Other

Let's return to clinical applications of the formula of repetition and its interruption: Emma grows aware of the active aspect of her sexuality, and Ka-Tzetnik stops repressing his own aggressive urges. We observe the clinical value of the subjective-active position when Emma sheds her phobia and Ka-Tzetnik stops suffering from insomnia. Judging by the therapeutic impact of subjectivization, acknowledgement of the drive by way of the subject's active positioning, we may assume that the roots of trauma inhere in the objectal-passive position. Lacan shows how drives, originating in the demand of the Other, are fundamentally passive, thereby consigning them to repetition. Consciousness acquired through analysis offers the small degree of choice the subject can attain by taking control over the drive and resisting it, or alternatively, to pursue it.

Inside the clinic and out, we can observe how drives originate in the demand of the Other. Saddam Hussein's father died when his mother was pregnant. She believed that the child she carried was a devil who killed his father. Did Saddam have any chance *not* to turn out monstrous when he grew up? A patient would suddenly fall asleep in the middle of the day. He told how his mother had raised him with the statement that "As a baby, when you were asleep you looked like a prince." How could he avoid falling asleep? Suicidal urges, too, can be the result of a subject's understanding that her conception was unwanted. Lacan's notion of "the demand of the other" is about "what I imagine the other expects from me." The human infant is, on the one hand, more dependent and helpless than any other young mammal, but on the other it is also more intelligent, calculating how to please and be loved by the other. This is how the drives evolve. They are a response aimed to survive the demand of the other as interpreted by the subject.

One interpretation of Lacan's well-known statement: "There is no sexual relationship" (Lacan 1998 p. 13) is that the relation is in language. Lacan disagreed with Strachey's translation of Freud's German *Trieb* with the

English *instinct* and proposed it should be *drive* instead. He saw Strachey's translation as a Freudian slip in its own right, caused by Strachey's biologistic bias. Lacan took up the project of psychoanalysis, which Freud had begun, with a clear wish for scientific approval, yet not at the price of a biologistic merging with psychiatry or neurology. The drive, unlike instinct, connotes the symbolic. Accepting Freud's approach, Lacan defined drive with reference to grammatical categories. The other formulates their demand in language, through its pre-existing channels, which also convey the response of the subject's drive.

Drives and Grammatical Structure

In his canonical formula, Lévi-Strauss showed the drive's passive as well as active tendencies. Going beyond Lévi-Strauss, Lacan pointed out how language affects the drives, as well as suggesting a third, reflexive position in relation to them. These three positions correspond with the three grammatical modes: active, passive, and what is called the middle position, reflexive. In the latter mode you could say that the subject actively occupies a passive role. Thus, for instance the three possible modes of the scopic drive are to see, to be seen, and to make oneself visible. While the subject usually is conscious of one aspect of the drive, the structural approach assumes that the drive always manifests in three dimensions. So, the sadistic person doesn't only dominate her or his victim, but is, also controlled by a guiding principle, some controlling idea or belief. The masochist conducts a ritual in which he or she surrenders control, and the fetishist identifies with the item substituting for the body, taking the position of an object by using one.

The main axis along which psychoanalysis moves, especially in its work with neurotic patients, is towards the manifestation or expression of the reflexive mode. The objective is for the patient to take as much responsibility as possible for the active way in which they pursue a passive position. The reflexive position is a form of ingenuousness – as if the subject were saying: It's not really me who is responsible for this desire, this drive. I'm merely its object. The analyst must present the demand of the other as interpreted by the subject, because if we were to point out "Look! It's your own interpretation, the outcome of your own desire!" we would be expecting from the ingenuous reflexive to acknowledge its own active position as a verb. The question is whether the other is really so demanding, or whether it serves conveniently so that we do not have to face the really hard question: "What in this demand do I desire?" Historically speaking, it may be that the subject had rigid parents with high expectations, but the subject also plays an active role maintaining the structure that exerts the demand.

What all this implies for our clinical work is that we must listen carefully to the patient's iterations of their narrative, with a view to small differences. How, for instance, this time they seem to be more actively involved as a subject. We may even look for a specific signal, something causing a noun in their narrative to turn into a verb, as in the illustration of the patient who would castigate himself for past failures by repeating: "I'm null and zero, null and zero, null and zero," and one day came up with the following statement: "I'm dialing back to zero, recalibrating: I'll take another look at everything I thought I knew till now and am open to see something new." In other words, he let go of the burden of the past to open a new page. He transformed noun into verb – a shift that embodies the transition from object to subject. We, psychoanalysts, want to capture this turnabout as it occurs, presenting the patient with their subjectivity as it shows up in their expression. Here's the subject in action. "You said it!" We think of the subject as one who refuses the repetition of non-presence. Repetition occurs when the same object re-appears. This exactly is the moment when we are there to draw attention: No, this time it's you!

The Rat Man and the Canonical Formula

Following Lévi-Strauss, Lacan applied the canonical formula to clinical cases, relating to dreams or symptoms. This is evident in his 1977 article "The Neurotic's Individual Myth" (Lacan 1977) in which he analyzed Freud's 1909 case of the Rat Man. Here I will consider how Lacan's analysis traces the drive as it evolves from passive to active.

As if possessed by a demon, Ernst Lanzer, better known as the Rat Man, felt pathologically driven to repeat an absurd scene in which he would acquit himself of a debt in a strangely roundabout manner. He was trying to return money he owed for a *pince-nez* to the officer who brought it to him, and the woman working in the post office who paid for them. It was in fact the latter person who paid on his behalf and not the officer, something the Rat Man knew. In the fantasy that compels him to act – even though he is aware it is a delusion – he must return the money to officer A, who will transfer it to another officer, who will pass it on to the postal clerk. Officer A appears in this myth because Lanzer met him during his reservist service, and the man told him a horrific story about a form of torture whereby a rat was made to enter the person's anus.

Restoring the Anal Object and Returning Debt in a Bid to Achieve Perfection

Lacan explained that the fantasy of a "rat in the anus" is a metaphor for the *wish for mythic perfection*. Here the body's topology (its various orifices) is deployed to render a wish for perfection. Similar to ancient myths featuring a primitive incestuous condition, here too the wish is to restore a lost primordial perfection.

Lanzer's associations, as described and analyzed in Freud's case study, help us understand how returning the debt, and applying a rat to a victim's anus become tied together in the figure of officer A, who in Lanzer's obsession was the addressee of the debt. The German for rat – *Rat* had become phonetically associated with the word *Spiel Ratten* – German for gambling money. Rats are associated with excrement – and since, in the unconscious, the release of excrement from the body equals castration, restoring the anal object to the body – which in the dream takes the shape of inserting rat into anus – signifies a return to perfection. Freud more commonly associated money and human waste. Another image in Lanzer's dream ties together paying back the debt, and recovering the anal object: that of the pince-nez covered with excrement. This image visually fuses together two signs that overlap with regard to money.

The different scenes of Lanzer's fantasies can be identified, like in the case of the natives: The anal phantasm of inserting rats into the anus represents how the scene of the body participates in Lanzer's private myth. Where in the scene of the body, the anal object must return to where it came from, in the social scene, the debt must be returned to the officer. Both actions seek to "stop the lack" and restore things to how they were. These scenes are connected by a shared signifier, namely the officer. The same officer who retailed the story about the rat in the anus, is also the officer to whom the debt must be returned.

The Son's Return of the Father's Debt

Freud observed that the irrational, compulsive urge to repay the officer for the pince-nez had emerged when Lanzer's parents forced him to marry a well-off woman rather than the poor woman he loved, repeating the father's act when he married a rich woman rather than the woman he loved.

Freud linked the Rat Man's bizarre behavior to two episodes from his father's life, which together made up the myth of the Rat Man's own birth. These reached the patient in his childhood and took the shape of a complaint voiced by his mother. His father, as mentioned, had married his mother for her money instead of the woman he really loved. The other story involved his father failing to return money he owed an officer who had paid for him. This acquittal of his father's debt by the son occurs in a number of images: returning money owed to an officer, putting back in its proper place the anal object as represented by the rat, as filling the lack represented by the body; and a hallucination in which his late father looks on while he masturbates. This may be a representation of the retentive position associated with masturbation functioning to heal the expulsivity in the conduct of a father who had financial debts.

Lacan refers to the case of the Rat Man in his above mentioned "The Neurotic's Individual Myth" (1977), to show how the iterative structure is consistent in private myth too. The father's debt repeats itself as the son's debt, causing Lanzer to develop his delusion of debt and guilt – like his father. Yet, unlike his father, he tries to counteract fate by paying back and restoring the father's image. Still, this doesn't afford the conditions for a normal existence. He is not allowed to succeed where his father failed. Until he resurrects his father's phallic honor, he is not free to pursue his own desires.

Here too the various scenes are interlinked. Since the Real father "carries" the Symbolic one, if the father is not in optimal condition, it puts the entire Symbolic order at risk. Often myth ties together ostensibly divergent scenes: In the Amazonian myth I mentioned earlier, for instance, if the lazy man allows his excrement to drop from the tree, the cosmic order will be upset with meteorites falling from the skies and destroying the land. The parallel of this catastrophe in the personal myth is the ruin of the Symbolic order in which the Rat Man lives. Given the link between worlds, the child will have to sacrifice himself to save the father, who is the stable core that holds the Symbolic order together. At issue, in Lanzer's case, is the myth of his own origins. Being the product of his father's dishonesty – financial as well as amorous – he must redeem his father so that the latter can, again, serve as the central axis of both familial and cosmic order. The same notion of the father as carrier of the Symbolic order can be traced back to the Papuan myth in which the tent's main joist has to pass through the father's back to ensure the safety of the tent, that is to say, the family.

Marrying Freud's Rich Daughter and Turnabout in the Myth

At some point Lanzer shares a thought with Freud concerning Freud's place in the transference. In his fantasy, he is annoyed with Freud who wants him to marry his rich daughter, something he feels he is compelled to agree with out of a sense of indebtedness, because Freud is treating him. This takes the following linguistic structure: Marrying Freud's rich daughter will be by way of paying back (verb) Lanzer's debt to his analyst. This payment will replace the debt (noun).

In his analysis of this case, Lacan employed the canonical formula. The passage from the first quaternary – just to remind – to its repetition in the second, helps embroider a myth that holds out a solution. With the Rat Man, the problem is his feelings of guilt about his father's transgressions, and the solution comes in the form of a myth which includes a difference, which is where reparation occurs. Here is how Lacan arranged the quaternaries in Lanzer's personal myth:

In the first quaternary, A standing for the father's debt, in relation to B – the officer in the military unit in which the father served, and the emotional debt to the poor woman whom the father did not marry, is analogous with how C, the son's debt, relates to officer D. The patient is obsessed with resolving his guilt by repeating and experiencing it and then trying to resolve it. The symptom will be dealt with by paying the debt to the military unit and to the poor woman, in their present representations, namely, by paying his debt to officer A and to the poor woman through marrying her. Psychoanalysis offers him a solution based on a change in the formula itself.

In the transference, Lanzer has a fantasy, which would seem mysterious and bizarre if we didn't know how to read it as myth: Freud offers him his rich daughter in marriage, and he cannot refuse because he feels he is indebted to Freud for everything he's done for him. Here is where the about-face occurs, at H:

> In the second quaternary E – the father's **debt** to F – the officer, and the poor woman, is analogous to G – Lanzer's feeling he must **pay** Freud by H – marrying the rich woman.

The first quaternary's equation of meaning stipulates that marrying a poor woman is like repaying the father's debt. In the repetition that constitutes the transference toward Freud, instead of feeling impelled to marry a poor woman to repay the father's debt, Lanzer feels obligated to marry a rich woman. The negative value of "poor woman" thus flips into the positive value of "rich woman," while the noun "debt" turns into an act of remuneration. The difference lies in the shift from passive to active, from noun to verb. The word "to pay" is a verb substituting for the noun "debt." It's important to note that at issue, rather than the subject's desire for a woman, is his desire to rid himself of his father's debt.

To conclude, we consistently see that the interruption that breaks repetition occurs in the transition from a negatively charged noun to a verb with a positive connotation through which the subject emerges as present. We can see this happening, in Emma's case, in the move from sexual object in the negative sense, to being a sexual subject in the positive sense; we see it, again, in the move from the evil goatsucker bird to the ovenbird's act of *ovenbirding* or – in the clinical vignette I mentioned above, from the bad "zero and nothing" to its positive counterpart in the act of starting afresh with a clean slate, and finally, in the case of the Rat Man when bad debt turns into good repayment. Clinical attention to these patterns is of importance because it enables us to make visible and accessible to patients their subjectivity whenever it emerges through repetition.

References

Dinur, Y. (K. Tsetnik). (1987). *Tzofen Edmah: The core journey of Auschwitz* [in Hebrew]. Hakibbutz Hameuchad.

Freud, S. (1909). Notes upon a case of an obsessional neurosis (The "Rat Man"). In *The standard edition* (Vol. 10, pp. 151–245). Hogarth Press.

Freud, S. (1953). A project for a scientific psychology (J. Strachey, Ed. & Trans.). *The standard edition of the complete psychological works of Sigmund Freud* (Vol. 1, pp. 283–397). Hogarth Press.

Lacan, J. (1977). *The neurotic's individual myth.* In J. Lacan (A. Sheridan, Trans.), *Ecrits; A selection* (pp. 111–147). W. W. Norton & Company.

Levi-Strauss, C. (1988) *The jealous potter* (trans. B. Chorier). University of Chicago.

Lacan, J. (1998). *The seminar of Jacques Lacan, Book XX: Encore, 1972–1973* (B. Fink, Trans.). W. W. Norton.

Chapter 11

Beyond Structure

Yehuda Israely

We have seen how language-based human behaviors were at the focus of Lévi-Strauss's scholarly interest. And yet he also looked at what is not given to symbolization, namely, the Real. Reference to this can be found in his introduction to Marcel Mauss's work, where he addresses the question of the signified that has no signifier. He calls it the "unthinkable" and does not discuss it explicitly. Psychoanalysts and anthropologists are propelled by different passions. Anthropologists don't consider what pre-exists or falls outside structure as an object of study. In this they are unlike psychoanalysts; they are not concerned with alleviating suffering of non-belonging.

Fu dwelled on the cusp of the structure. He was the village fool of Matroku, a village belonging to the Bobo tribe in Burkina Faso in west Africa. He didn't speak, his hair was netted and dirty, and it was obvious he had not washed or changed the rags in which he dressed for a long time. He'd limp along the path that surrounded the village, dividing between it and the forest.

Fu garbled meaningless sounds. He constantly put his hand on his backside and smelled it. Children would run after him, calling, "Fu! Fu!" He would scare them, chasing them away with his walking stick, but soon, magnetized, they would return to tag behind him. Fu existed on the line – both in the real, actual sense, by constantly circling the village's perimeter path rather than withdrawing into the forest, as well as metaphorically, while not participating in the social discourse, he stayed in touch with the community.

People like Fu are not amenable to structure and stay attached to the object. Fu doesn't let go of the object, in his case, the anal object: he doesn't talk, he doesn't participate in the order of symbols that replace the object. The same goes for the myth about the two brothers-in-law who went out in search of parrot feathers for the wedding, mentioned in Chapter 4 with reference to kinship relations. The brother-in-law who did not give away his sister at the wedding ceremony refused to let go of the anal object. This is how he ended up outside the system, locked in an auto-erotic cycle, as he sat in a tree, consuming his own excrement.

Lévi-Strauss, unlike Freud and Lacan, had no therapeutic ambitions. Unlike the analytic subject, the community the anthropologist studies has no body and

DOI: 10.4324/9781003773764-12

isn't an actual organism. When the subject's *jouissance* does not agree with social structure, they seek out the psychoanalyst for help with the suffering this generates. The anthropologist does not countenance this. Subjects who elude language, says Lévi-Strauss, he therefore leaves to the psychoanalysts.

One way to distinguish between people is between those who manage to live in the structure and thrive in it, and those who don't. Both groups have important cultural roles, since those who have more difficulty adjusting themselves to the structure often help it evolve, thereby affecting the entire community. Like Freud, who defines neurosis as a reaction to civilization's demand for the repression of our instincts, Lévi-Strauss defines phenomena like spirit possession as occurring to those who are more sensitive to the inconsistencies and paradoxes of the symbolic system.

The native person who is sick challenges the shaman to expand the tribe's symbolic frame and enable changes in meanings that cause suffering. The shaman can achieve such shifts in meaning either by inventing another myth or by adjusting existing ones, offering a way out through the myth's narrative. An interesting instance of the first option – creating a new myth in the face of a new crisis – appears in the 16th century Kabbalist mysticism of Rabbi Isaac Luria of Safed. The mystical Kabbalist principle of *tsimtsum* (withdrawal or contraction) describes God's withdrawal of his own infinity to make space for creating the world and humans. In so doing God gave humans power and space to affect their own fate. The origins of this myth have been traced back to the Jews' expulsion from Spain in 1492, and it is interesting to consider how in that context the myth would have served the Jews to come to terms with this historical event, turning it into something less catastrophic and more bearable. Lack and fragmentation are intrinsic parts of the divinity (Scholem 1946).

Sometimes, nevertheless, the structure cannot be expanded to make possible inclusion in the symbolic narrative. These states are beyond language and myth. The Real may manifest in pathological conditions: originating beyond language it takes the shape of psychosis. Under the onslaught of the Real, there is no point in reaching for a presumably shared myth or trauma.

But the Real appears not only in pathology. For the shaman, as well as the mystic and the psychoanalyst, a consciously appointed position exists outside the symbolic order. From this position change from outside, into the patient's symbolic domain, can be introduced. To alter the story, one must recognize the nature of the story as such, which is to say, one must have a footing extraneous to it.

Schreber's Psychosis and Loss of Faith in the Symbol

What happens when the psychotic person encounters the structure represented by language? Or maybe we should first turn to an even more fundamental question: what does it take for a person to be willing to live in language, and does a person choose their own psychic structure?

Lacan believes it involves unconscious choice, a gamble: do we trust the symbol or don't we? Since it is engaged unconsciously, the subject carries no responsibility for the choice. Lacan (1973–1974) compares it to Pascal's famous wager about the existence of God. Pascal argues that the wager is made on the basis of an assessment of gain: it's worth one's while to believe in God. This is how he explains it: if God exists, and we decide to believe, then we will have gained eternal life, while someone who does not, will go to Hell. If, on the other hand, we put our bets on faith though God doesn't exist, there's no harm done; we have merely wasted our time observing religious rules – not much of a loss, at least in Pascal's eyes. Lacan's big question concerns the existence of the human subject rather than of God, and his answer to Pascal's question is, "I wager, therefore I am" – exist, that is, as a subject. The big Other, for Lacan, on whom we put our bets is language, rather than God. In putting their faith in language representing reality, and by being willing to enter language, subjects turn themselves into narrative creatures, which is to say: subjects. People suffering from psychosis, by contrast, fail to wager on language, which leaves them outside reality, unable to exist as subjects.

Those who cannot enter into structure, and do not put their trust in the signifier, constitute what Lévi-Strauss called the "signified without signifier." In 1903 Daniel Schreber wrote a book about his psychotic experiences, which Freud studied and discussed extensively. His difficulty in living within the structures of language manifested itself early on when he fell victim to hypochondria, as the inherent lack of signifiers came to take the form of being unable to get a diagnosis for actual physical complaints. Schreber's psychotic episode was triggered by two life events that happened to coincide and somehow contradict, something he was unable to mentally accommodate. On the one hand, he and his wife had learned they could not have children, that he could not take the paternal function, while, on the other, he was appointed as presiding judge of a higher court of justice, a position of high authority.

Comparing Helen Keller and Daniel Schreber, or Opposite Processes: Loss of the Signifier and Its Discovery

Assuming that in psychosis the signified goes without signifier, in the case of the hypochondria that was the first harbinger of Schreber's psychotic breakdown, what was missing was a diagnosis for his physical complaints; there were no signifiers for the signified which was Schreber-as-a-body. What he subjectively experienced as the body's falling apart, was nothing but a deterioration of Schreber's ability to symbolize the body. Here the body can be seen as a metaphoric setting of the mind, in this case: of a dissolving symbolic structure. By contrast, looking back at Chapter 2, and its discussion of the myth of the subject's emergence in the case of Helen Keller, we see the opposite taking place: the discovery of the signifier as it joins the signified.

What was it that emerged in Helen Keller when she encountered the word, the signifier? An experience of lack was triggered, leading to the ability to crave and to feel. Once she experienced membership in a world made up of words, she felt all nameable things around her coming to life in language. A mirror image of the ecstasy of this moment, is that of Schreber's ruin when his symbolic structure crumbled. The absence of lack associated with the absence of symbolic order is apparent in Schreber's psychotic vision about the removal of suffering from the world. The messianic drive comes to cover up the lack of symbolic order Closing over or being filled, as it were, absence re-appears in the vocation of the person who is set to resolve what's lacking in the world. Schreber recounts how he loses vital power, a process mediated through the loss of bodily parts – he loses his stomach, his lungs – while he goes on living. These are concrete images for symbolic castration, but they do not evolve beyond the imaginary dimension.

Another way Schreber has of translating symbolic to imaginary, is by the compromised grid of signification taking on the visual shape of cosmic radiation, a kind of extension of the neural network that bestows meaning on everything he fails to grasp due to his psychosis. Schreber's psychotic vision is that all humans emit such cosmic radiation, yet while in the case of ordinary people, after death, this web dissolves, with well-known figures like Bismarck or Goethe it remains intact. This element of Schreber's vision – the survival of the symbolic name through the figure of actual rays, confirms the idea that these are concrete representations of signifiers. The signifier survives the organism as part of the culture, even in Schreber's psychotic vision.

The signifying elements manifest themselves in Schreber's text similar to how they do among Amazonian natives or in the case of little Hans. Schreber, too, worries about the phallus and its loss; he is troubled by secretions as well – in the form of images of God eviscerating him, and other unconscious raw materials. Unlike Hans or the natives, however, signifying elements, in his case, are not really signifiers. They do not amount to a meaning-making structure; a mythic narrative including chains of meanings. What appears as a message with a faulty code, is a message about a faulty code. It may even be more accurate to say it is no message at all, but a faulty code laid bare because the message-bearing subject has vanished.

Paranoia – Threat of the Subject's Elimination

After hypochondria, Schreber was visited by paranoia. Under paranoia the subject stands to be eliminated due to the dissolution of the symbolic system that normally sustains it. Paranoid delusions took the place of the common myths with which Schreber lived until then. Now Schreber called his psychiatrist, Dr Flechsig, a "soul murderer," casting him as the cause for his loss of subjectivity. The surrounding world, stripped of signifiers, is drained of vitality and people now appear as zombies: soulless. When the connection between signifier and signified collapses – exactly the opposite of Helen Keller's experience – libido leaches away from the world and inward, leaving everything outside lifeless. This is when dystopian images come into play, like: "the end of the world is nigh" – unless Schreber acts to save it. Schreber, in Lévi-Straussian terms, has stopped participating in exchange relations. The same would be true of states of catatonia, melancholy, erotomania, and paranoia. "Leave me alone," expresses the paranoid patient's one desire.

Being God's Wife – Loss of the Phallic Signifier

While the comparison between Schreber and Helen Keller shows us how the signifier she discovered, imbuing her with life, is the same signifier Schreber lost and made him experience loss of life; the comparison between Schreber and little Hans bears out that the lost basic signifier of vitality was the phallic signifier. In his paranoid phase, Schreber came to see Flechsig as threatening to rape him. This erotomaniac idea evolved into Schreber's later belief that he was God's wife. Freud interpreted this as a feminine homosexual identification which communicates submission in the face of the father, the rivalry with whom Schreber presumably was denying. Lacan, however, drew attention to the absent phallus in Schreber's paranoia, which was rendered through both the feminine position Schreber chose to occupy, and the imagery around getting a phallus in the form of the sexual encounter with Dr Flechsig. Here is Schreber's missing signifier. In Chapter 9, when discussing little Hans and animism, we saw Hans used the phallus as an animistic signifier. We can say the same of Schreber, except that in his case we observe that the emptying of animism, the removal of a vitality earlier associated with the world, goes hand in hand with loss of the phallic. Lacan did not explain Schreber's self-identification as the wife of God, or the feeling he shared with Freud that it "would be nice to be a woman," as evidence of a homosexual tendency or feminine cravings, but rather saw it as an attempt to give meaning to the loss of the organ of meaning, which is no other than the phallic signifier. For Lacan, Schreber's female identification was a way of deploying the body to render the subject's lack of a signifier. The fantasy of being penetrated by God's phallus is his way of wishing for the signifier to restore his psyche. The fantasy, however, does not evolve beyond imaginary figures.

Being the Phallus – Being the Origin of the World

In Schreber's psychotic vision, he would bring about the onset of a new humanity. In neurosis, the phallus remains lacking, however much the individual decries this. Zhuangzi, who was mentioned in Chapter 5, on totemism, dreamt he was a butterfly, and on waking could not tell whether he was a butterfly dreaming he was Zhuangzi. Zhuangzi's doubt whether his shape represented him is a defense against psychotic phallic identification. If this was a case of psychosis, Zhuangzi would not have been vulnerable to this doubt. The psychotic subject's figure is what it is in the Other's gaze. If their language system was functional, they could have had an identity based on a signifier in a signifying network. They could have been represented as a subject in relation to other subjects who, in their turn, are represented by signifiers. The psychotic person's participation in this grid is compromised, so their identity must rely on the imaginary dimension, where it is subject to the gaze of the Other. Rather than being "part of the symbolic fabric" it is "subject to the Other's gaze." This is their identity. This is how they become a "thing."

Psychosis involves a loss in symbolizing ability. For Schreber, the loss of the phallic, in the sense of signification, assumes the imaginary form of feminization with regard to his own body, and of catastrophe where it concerns the world. To fix his own castration, which is attributed to the world, Schreber must become the world's lacking phallus and thus restore perfection. Being "the wife of God" is to be the world's missing phallus, so essentially, he is the solution to what is missing in God, the world, and the Other.

The phallus is the signifier of signification. As in the case of Hans, it is attributed to whoever participates in language (Lacan 1998). In Schreber's vision, he himself is the primary, phallic signifier on whose basis the collapsed symbolic world was created. Why does his identification as the wife of God show him to be taking the position of the phallus? In what equation is phallus analogical to woman? This equation ties together three scenes of lack in the effort to formulate a myth of the resurrection of the symbolic order. Even as the phallus may be absent, so that its presence is the image of perfection on the scene of the body, a wife can be what God misses, and Schreber's presence in that feminine form is the image of religious perfection.

For Schreber, the metaphor of the wife who complements God serves as an image of the return of the missing signifier. The imaginary figure, however, does not achieve the status of signifier. And in the absence of this signifier, Schreber describes how, having lost vitality, he feels like a corpse, excrement, a chunk of meat – something that threatens to befall the whole of humanity at the end of the world. This is apparent in his delusion where God's cosmic rays take control of his intestines, pushing out his excrement. At the same time, he feels how God takes away his vital power, leaving him a corpse. By his own interpretation, Schreber considers himself an idiot who can no longer control his discharges. This is how he renders himself account of the link between the absent signifier and his body's dissolution (Freud 1958).

Trauma as Undoing Structure, and the Healing Shift from Passive to Active

In Chapter 10's discussion of Lévi-Strauss's elaboration on Freud's notion of traumatic repetition, there is the moment when noun turns into verb, and passive becomes active. In that Chapter's reference to the case of Emma,

Freud identified the repetitive nature of trauma. Emma made the transition from sexual object at age eight to being subject to sexual attraction at age 12. It was, in effect, only with the emergence of subjecthood – an active stance vis-à-vis the sex drive – that it became possible for her to see that at her younger age, trauma involved an appropriation of subjecthood, making her the object of another person's drive. That the transition to activity has a healing effect indicates traumatic injury is to subjecthood itself: a person's status as craving and making choices. If psychotic individuals lack the mythic mechanisms that maintain them as subjects within a grid of signifiers and images, trauma has the power to break up this structure in neurotic people. An especially graphic illustration would be the scene of a suicide bombing scattered with mutilated bodies: here the myth of body integrity crashes and along with it, the subject.

Trauma is followed by dissociation, which itself constitutes another step away from participation in the symbolic domain supporting subjecthood. Trauma causes people to shrink and withdraw from the world, shedding parts of the narrative from which they have become detached. Emma does not want to admit into her life such threatening signifiers as "laughter," "clothes," or "being alone in a shop." The dissociative processes underlying her self-restraint are evident. Such processes can be observed not only in extreme conditions like complex post-trauma. At different intensities, they manifest on a dissociative sequence – from personality disorder down to a sense of reduced value of the world outside. Trauma, like psychosis, with its dissociative response, is experienced as evacuation of the libido invested in the world. This takes the inverse direction from the animistic experience Helen Keller describes. When words appear, the subject comes to life and gets connected to the world, while in the case of trauma, loss of trust in words together with withdrawal from the world damages the subject's sense of being and being present in their life.

While we treat words as what sustains subjects' being, they may in fact also be crushed by signifiers. When do signifiers support, and when do they undermine subjecthood? The answer to this question can be found in the repetitious nature of the canonical formulation, which is to say, in the earlier mentioned shift from passive object to active subject. Experience is narrowly tied to the subject's relation to language: when subjects take the position of the speaker they can heal the traumatic experience of being "spoken-about" objects, when it is others who determine who they are.

This is the thought behind trauma therapy: the therapist's close listening encourages the patient to talk about their trauma. In doing so, the patient reformulates the myth of their own life, turning it into a narrative while also taking the position of the speaker. A speaker who articulates her or his own being, featuring in their own myth of creation.

Lacan refers to Hamlet when he discusses the question of being. When Hamlet asks himself whether to be or not to be, Lacan hears: To be or not to be a speaker? The choice is between being passive, the one who is spoken about, the mother's object, lacking any footing for agency, or to be an active speaker who is the subject of his own myth of creation, taking a role in the family myth in which he is fated to belong, and avenge his father's death.

The Shaman – Between Symbolic and Real

In his book *White Doctor, Black Gods* (2006), Dr Ori Schwartzman, a psychiatrist, writes about his insights concerning differences in western and native African attitudes to psychosis. Male and female shamans are identified in childhood on the basis of features that in western terminology would be described as hallucinatory tendencies, like seizures, suggesting their ability to enter a trance, or dissociative symptoms indicating that they have an ability to dwell in different worlds or to lend their bodies to spirits and demons. These children communicate with spirits and demons, and the shamans who are their enthusiastic mentors stimulate them to develop these features.

Animistic ways of thinking, which attribute a soul to every existing thing, exclude the possibility of random events. Every illness has a reason tying it to someone's intention: it may be a human enemy who cast a spell; the spirit of the antelope who takes revenge after its life was taken without due thanks, or the revenge of the ancestors who have been neglected in rituals and sacrifices. The native fills perplexity with animistic explanations, much like the western individual uses science and religion.

Schwartzman writes about a tribal chief whom he diagnosed as suffering with delusional schizophrenia, with hallucinations and cognitive decline, whose social prestige only grew as these symptoms increased. Villagers saw the chief as enlightened, a prophet and channel for divine voices. In the space native culture gives to the imagination, which in western eyes would seem delusional, the distinction between faith and pathology blurs. This lack of distinction has positive sides: Native cultures generally assume the subject is not to blame for the sickness from which they suffer. They are possessed by a demon who must be exorcised, and so neuroses, with their typical sense of conflict and guilt, are less common. They are also socially much more accepted and rehabilitated than in the west. They are not labelled as "sick," carrying a "schizophrenic" identity. Anyone can be exposed to demons.

From the shaman's perspective, what makes the patient's delusions and hallucinations pathological, is the extent to which the latter suffers from them – not the fact that they occur. The demon attacks the patient and takes them into a spirit world against their will; the shaman, by contrast, intentionally enters a trance so the ancestral spirits will visit her or him, using him as a conduit for fighting the demons. While the patient does not intend to enter a trance, the physician does so on their own initiative, since it is from here they derive their healing power.

The shaman is picked for this task from early childhood, due to his or her proximity to domains beyond reality. Like Fu, the village idiot, who metaphorically traces the limits of culture by walking up and down the path that separates village from forest, the shaman treads the line between Symbolic and Real, between cultural and wild. Unlike the village idiot, however, the shaman has the ability to participate in the social order and give meaning to common myths.

People with magical powers don't necessarily take them from the same sources. Schwartzman explains that healers associated with the community's leadership have a connection with ancestral spirits, and through them with the community gods. Independent witches, by contrast, who wield evil powers, are associated with the natural forces often considered to be behind the suffering of the sick. Healers, then, are associated with the community's Symbolic order, and witches with what's beyond it: the animal, pre-human, which myth identifies with regressive behavior, and autoerotic withdrawal into the self. These witches are ascribed regressive activities of the kind we are familiar with from myth: incest, bestiality, coprophagy, and cannibalism. Often, witches are considered the offspring of incestuous relations. The native perspective on this is that these witches' regressive behaviors occur in the mythical, spiritual parallel world, not in actual, here and now life.

Psychoanalysis as Magic, the Analyst as Shaman

In his 1963 article, "The Sorcerer and his Magic," Lévi-Strauss explains the workings of magic. In the case of a spell, for instance, socially ostracizing a person, though, say, voodoo magic, the community ousts her or him, so that the person is cut off from the usual components of their identity in the social-symbolic domain. This almost inevitably causes such great fear it even compromises their physiological reactions, threatening their life.

From a non-essentialist, structuralist viewpoint like Lévi-Strauss's, and even more so from Lacan's postmodern perspective, reality is generated by myth. There is no other reality. If a man lives within a voodoo myth in which a spell has been put on him, fear will eventually kill him, and this will then further bolster the community's system of beliefs. For witchcraft to work – and the same goes for the opposite power of healing – two essential conditions must be obtained in the structure that is reality. One is an intergenerationally transmitted tradition with inner coherence. Tradition comes under the community's responsibility. The second condition is the creativity of the shaman tasked with inventing and applying methods of healing, and with "embroidering" stories and myths for people and problems. These conditions occur in both the native tribe and the psychoanalytic discourse in both the shaman's and the psychoanalyst's therapeutic approach. The various schools of psychoanalysis have their traditional ways of passing on knowledge, as well as the setting's rituals and ceremonies regarding money, time, communication outside the clinic, and so on. Often analysands are psychoanalysts themselves, and the mythic jargon is a shared mythic element of the community. As Freud indicated, however, every analytic treatment is a new and unique invention for the patient in question.

Freud and Lacan were well aware that therapies for the psyche did not begin with the emergence of psychoanalysis. The unconscious and language had been brought to bear in the treatment of the psyche before Freud formulated psychoanalytic theory. The Iroquois who live on the North American plains believe that in addition to their conscious wishes, dreams tell them about wishes they don't know they have; it is their belief that they therefore must try to fulfil their wishes as they manifest in their dreams (Wallace 1958). They are helped in this by "psychoanalytic" fellow tribal people who are more expert than others in understanding what wish a certain dream expresses. Though the theoretical formulation of psychoanalytic healing only began with Freud, its mythic formulation was being used as a healing method even in the remote past.

From a different angle, we can look at psychoanalysis as a type of magic, too. Freud mentions that a simple person might think of the effects of psychoanalysis as magic, something he himself calls "slow magic" (1926). We might ask again how the talking cure can heal. Because humans live in the domain of signifiers, they will be affected – for better and for worse – by the words they use. Lacan, the postmodernist, emphasized this even more than did Freud and Lévi-Strauss. Both psychoanalyst and shaman rely on the power of words. To the extent that we live (in) a story, alterations to that story will have actual, bodily consequences. In the case of Lacan, this is the essence of psychoanalysis; to use symbolic means to effect concrete, real change.

One way in which the shaman and psychoanalyst are alike is that both use the fact that the patient believes they have knowledge, even though they themselves know they don't. This ascription of knowledge serves to ground faith in knowledge as such; if there are people who know, then there must be knowledge. Knowledge is the parallel metaphoric system – whether analytic concepts, or demons and spirits – that bring about parallel change in the patient's mind. Like the shaman who is situated on the margins of the Symbolic order, the psychoanalyst is positioned outside the mythic reality from which it is possible to dissolve, reconstruct, and change things in the individual's myth of creation. Lacan says that though we tell our patients to bring up anything that comes to mind, we must always remember that these are only words. Because we also know how to place ourselves outside words, we occupy the Archimedean position that allows us to enable change in a symbolic reality.

The triumph of faith and structure over reason is manifest in a story Lévi-Strauss included in a chapter on witches and spells in his *Structural Anthropology* (Lévi-Strauss 1963); it derives from a collection of folk tales of the New Mexico Zuni tribe (Cushing 1901).

At the risk of being put to death, even though he knew he wasn't at fault, an unfortunate young man found himself confessing he had been using magic powers. In some weird way, he even believed it himself, though he knew he had not intended to put the girl under a spell. True, he had grabbed her by the arm, but with no harmful intention. He could not have known she would experience a hysterical fit and pass out. To appear less guilty, he argued the magic power had meanwhile left him – even though he had never had such power to begin with. The investigation staged by the shamans was never aimed to reveal the truth. Much like the practices of the Inquisition, it came to claim and confirm tribal beliefs. This was why he gave them what they wanted. Moreover, he himself shared the tribes' beliefs and considered himself guilty. He offered them a version of the events that confirmed the community's magical way of thinking – something in which he also took part.

What is the secret power of the analyst and the shaman, if not their knowledge? Well, in contrast to what might be expected, the answer is actually their lack of knowledge. What the shaman and the analyst do know is what to do so that knowledge operates through them. They know how to step aside, or enter a trance, not because they know how to direct the healing, but because they know how to position themselves in order to participate in a process that has its own movement. These are the transference relations in the broad sense. Transference includes not only the patient's feelings toward the therapist, but the entire symbolic world that the analysand brings into the clinic, and the analyst has no choice but to surrender to their role within this structure. Surrendering to the transference relationship is one form of surrendering to the world, and therefore analysts have something to learn from mystics.

Mysticism – Dissolving the Boundaries of the Self and Merging with the World

Mysticism is relevant here because, in western monotheistic cultures, as in literate eastern ones, it has come to replace the shamanism of tribal cultures; all are liminal phenomena exceeding the domain of verbal expression. Both shaman, mystic and psychoanalyst, work with trance, offering themselves to something that operates through them. These can be animistic powers in the case of the shaman; divine presence in that of the mystic, or an unconsciously generated act, in the case of the psychoanalyst.

We have mentioned that people with a psychotic structure lost their grip on conventional signifying relations between things. They have a hard time participating in shared myth and living by the meanings it generates. This state of mind, into which the psychotic person is locked, is precisely what the mystic wants to reach, but with this difference: the psychotic person has been cast out from language, which has crumbled. Schreber's case is illustrative: he is left with a dismembered body, unable to sustain himself in the myth of his work as a jurist. Mystics however actively deploy language to enter an ecstatic experience that then takes them beyond words.

The person who suffers from psychosis, because language, for them, has fallen apart, withdraws into him or herself, investing their libido there. Mystics, by contrast, deploy culture, using text, music, and movement to sustain a myth in which they are part of the created world. So, when a mystic, say a whirling dervish, uses the body, it's part of symbolic rites. While psychotics turn inward, mystics direct themselves outwards: the former's inner world evacuates due to language's vanishing; the latter's fills because they move beyond language. This is the mystical-animistic experience Keller had when she realized everything had a name and she was part of a symbolic grid. Keller (1903) reports on her direct relationship with the world in a manner that reminds of mystic ecstasy. Mystics, like shamans, are protected from psychosis by a firm hold in the Symbolic order. In the past, Jewish mysticism, Kabbala, was open to study only to those who were forty years and older; only once the student has become solidly rooted in the Symbolic. Often mystics, like shamans, also practice healing. Both approaches set great store by ecstatic experience and both strive for transformation, of healer and patient. This is achieved through ceremonies and rituals that facilitate union with higher powers, like gods. The magical mysticism called "practical mysticism" is fully a shamanic practice – including amulets and exorcism. Theoretical mysticism, on the other hand, has no interest in affecting the world: it seeks to influence the mystic's psyche. The mystic seeks to be one with God or creation, to surrender to something larger than themselves and shed the illusion of a separate, autonomous ego.

Theoretical mysticism, shamanism and psychoanalysis interlink through their shared experience of trance – the annulment of detached identity. Ecstatic experience is reached via different routes. Sufi dervishes achieve it through dance; archers by surrendering to something inside that chooses when to release the arrow; Jewish mystics in the Abulafian tradition attain self-transcendence by meditating on the holy letters of God's name; while yogi practice breathing. Today, in western societies, there is a rise in the use of consciousness altering substances, of the kind shamans worldwide have drawn on in their search for mystical-animistic experiences cancelling out the ego's boundaries to become directly absorbed in the created world.

References

[שוורצמן, א.[2007] רופא לבן אלים שחורים. אריה ניר Shwartzman, U. (2007) *White doctor, black gods.* Arye Nir Pub. (In Hebrew)

Cushing, F. H. (1901). *Zuni Folk Tales.* G.P. Putnam's Sons.

Freud, S. (1926). A question of lay analysis. In J. Strachey (Ed. and Trans.), *The standard edition of the complete psychological works of Sigmund Freud* (Vol. 20, pp. 177–258). Hogarth Press.

Freud, S. (1958). Psycho-analytic notes on an autobiographical account of a case of paranoia (Dementia paranoides). In J. Strachey (Ed. & Trans.), *The standard edition of the complete psychological works of Sigmund Freud* (Vol. 12, pp. 1–82). Hogarth Press. (Original work published 1911.)

Keller, H. (1903). *The story of my life.* Doubleday, Page & Company.

Lacan, J. (1973–1974). *Seminar XVI – From one other to the other* (C. Gallagher, Trans.) Unpublished manuscript.

Lacan, J. (1998). *The seminar of Jacques Lacan, Book XX: Encore* (B. Fink, Trans.). W. W. Norton & Company.

Lévi-Strauss, C. (1963). The sorcerer and his magic. In *Structural anthropology.* Basic Books.

Scholem, G. (1971). *The Messianic idea in Kabbalah* (trans. M. M. Meyer). Schocken Books. (Original work published in Hebrew 1971.)

Scholem, G. (1946). *Major trends in Jewish mysticism.* Schocken Books.

Schreber, D. P. (1903). *Memoirs of my nervous illness.* New York Review of Books.

Schwartzman, O. (2006). *White doctor, black gods.* Aryeh Nir (in Hebrew).

Wallace, A. F. C. (1958). Dreams and the wishes of the soul: A type of psychoanalytic theory among the seventeenth century Iroquois. *American Anthropologist*, 60(2), 234–246.

Chapter 12

The Clinic of the Real

Yehuda Israely

Up to this point, the book has moved along a single axis: how human beings exist within structures of language: myths, narratives, turns of phrase, and formulas of meaning, and how the clinic of the Symbolic can hold a subject inside a web of signification that sustains him. Yet it is precisely this work that reveals an inner limit of structure; not everything that drives the subject can be translated, and not everything that repeats yields to interpretation. Language leaves a remainder that is not "more meaning," but rather a letter, a sound, a point of enjoyment, something that insists beyond the network, and can expose the symbolic network as a defense against this enjoyment. This is why the final chapter does not come to cancel the earlier ones, but to perform a subversion upon them, to show that structure was a pre-condition; that only after meaning has been built can one hear what does not enter meaning and that this is where the Real Unconscious begins. It comes with ethics that seek a certain distance from the Other and from the knowledge attributed to it.

The orientation of the cure in the clinic of the Symbolic continues the ethics implied by the Indigenous cultures Lévi-Strauss studied, to be woven into culture. Accordingly, the aim of treatment is to sustain the subject within his myths. It is there that the subject exists between the signifiers of the narratives and the myths of his singular fate. All this remains true for Lacan until the moment he makes his turn from the clinic of the Symbolic to the clinic of the Real.

In this chapter, I propose to understand Lacan's late turn not as the replacement of one clinic by another, but as a shift of center of gravity, from meaning and belonging to knotting and enjoyment, from an interpretation that adds knowledge to an operation that undermines the status of knowledge, from a subject who exists in a myth to a "speaking being" that is bound to its sinthome. There is clinical value in crossing the limits of the Symbolic clinic, through the layers of listening, to the Real unconscious, and finally to topology, act, and ethics, to clarify what I will call a clinic of subversion.

This change grows out of analytic experience. Lacan expresses dissatisfaction with the limit of the Symbolic clinic's power to cure. It is certainly a way of working with a patient that can relieve suffering, giving it sense; yet Lacan encounters the same blockage, the same dissatisfaction, that pushed Freud to

DOI: 10.4324/9781003773764-13

write *Beyond the Pleasure Principle*. For Freud as well, recollection and the construction of a narrative, whose power he initially believed in deeply, did not suffice to overcome the death drive in its many forms: masochism, the negative therapeutic reaction, or trauma. They ran up against the impotence of the Symbolic clinic, the clinic of meaning.

Among Lacanians, the clinic of the Real was so innovative that it often eclipsed the achievements of early Lacan, who forged an integration of Freud and Lévi-Strauss. One of the aims of this book is to return the Symbolic clinic to psychoanalysis. There is still immense value in construction and interpretation: in the patient's need to belong to social orders, to matter to those around him, to belong to the myths that sustain him as a subject. A deep engagement with Freud and Lévi-Strauss remains essential to the analyst's training. In work with psychosis, the clinic can function as scaffolding for the patient's structural life; and in work with trauma, as Lacan puts it, the aim is to turn trauma into tragedy, into something that can be articulated, and to reach a kind of reconciliation through the structure of drama, up to its tragic resolution.

Often, it's not enough, but understanding how the structures of language operate upon the subject matters even when one's aim is to go beyond language. The clinical ethics of late Lacan seeks a certain release from symbolic structures, to open a space between the speaking being and the language that comes from the Other and constructs him as a subject. In fact, the clinic of the Real treats the clinic of the Symbolic itself as a symptom. That is to say: it is not only the patient who produces a symptom; our own attachment to meaning can become symptomatic, a way of not touching jouissance. This is where late Lacan's suspicion appears; the Symbolic does not only organize the subject, at times the insistence on meaning itself becomes a defense. One can therefore say that the clinic of the Real treats the clinic of the Symbolic as a symptom: it asks when "sense" is serving as a way of not coming up against enjoyment.

There is something to be gained beyond identification as a subject within a structure, and this is especially true of analysis as the training of an analyst. To change, or loosen something in the patient's narrative, the analyst must occupy a position that is, at least in part, outside the structure, from which the structure can be seen. One must know a great deal about how the Symbolic works to go, and to lead, beyond it.

Layers of Listening

A position that joins the clinic of the Symbolic with a clinic that goes beyond the Symbolic is expressed in a remark Lacan makes about himself, one he recommends to other analysts as well: to be a poem. "I am not a poet, I am a poem, a poem that is written, even if it looks like a subject" (Lacan ([1964–1965] 1977, p. viii). Does it mean to speak poetry as if one were a poet? No, not a poet, but a poem. Perhaps to be, oneself, like a poem: structured like a poem, to have the effect of a poem. What is it, in a poem, that should characterize the analyst's position? His way of listening?

Beyond the sense of the words? "Being a poem" is not a matter of beauty or inspiration, but of listening: hearing in speech not only meaning, but also repetition, sound, a cut, and the solitary letter that carries jouissance.

What is said in the patient's free associations can be heard as belonging to different strata of structure, from the most abstract level of the Symbolic order, the shared myth, down to the concrete, Real level of sound, with its singular importance. To be a poem is to listen to all the layers of language contained in a poem, including the Real, the particular, the sensuous, the incidental, the meaningless. There is a continuum between these poles. At the highest level of abstract complexity stands myth: a system of meanings alone. Myth is distilled sense, cleansed of sensory elements such as sound or rhyme, cleansed of the materiality of language. It is so abstract that it cannot be expressed except through a narrative, in which there is not only meaning. Pure myth is by definition translatable: it keeps its sense in any language, in any genre, and in any literary form.

A narrative begins with the ambition to tell the myth and ends by being only one more of the myth's versions. A narrative is harder to translate because it bears the character of the language and the medium in which it appears. Narrative versions of myth are constrained by the linearity of speech. Myth itself is synchronic in structure, not diachronic in narrative. Just as the signifier aims at the thing itself yet only translates itself into another signifier, so too the versions of a myth never stop missing the mark and calling for yet another version. The relation between narrative and myth is like that between demand and desire. Demand can be formulated; desire rises from its repetition. As demand gives form to desire and the ego gives form to the subject; so, narrative gives form to myth.

Narrative is made of tropes turns that carry meaning by making one thing stand in for another. These tropes are variations on a formula of meaning. According to that formula, we say that one thing is like another, and therefore it becomes knowable. In what way is A like B? Here we have different variations on the different senses of "like." Like, but... These are the tropes, the turns of phrase. Metaphor is "like, but otherwise"; metonymy is "like" without an added surplus of meaning; hyperbole says "like, but more"; synecdoche says "like, but partially"; and irony or cynicism says, "like but reversed." Turns of phrase can be invented without end.

Beneath the turns of phrase lies their ancestor: metaphor. This is the basic cell of meaning as Lévi-Strauss formulated it; the quartet in which there is an analogy between pairs of oppositions. This is the fundamental "like" that constitutes the formula of meaning in Lévi-Strauss: A is to B as C is to D. Red is to blue as sensitive is to indifferent.

The Real Unconscious

Up to this point, I have described the workings of the Symbolic unconscious, which is grounded in relations among signifiers. But language has two further aspects that belong to the Real unconscious. The first is the isolated signifier: because it is not tied to other signifiers, and does not appear in the quartets of meaning, in the signifying network, it is more accurate to call it a sign, or a letter, so as to mark its solitary character. The second aspect is sound, the sensory side of language. These two aspects of speech eventually point to jouissance: points to where one identifies with the unraveling of Imaginary-Symbolic, virtual identities.

The isolated signifier does not take part in the economy of exchange. It is an arbitrary, meaningless mark, like a letter that is not woven into a word. The isolated signifier does not represent meaning; it produces jouissance.

The isolated signifier belongs to the poem. A story, a narrative, exists only by virtue of the links between its signifiers, bound to one another through turns of phrase. Myth is made of layers of narratives piled one upon another in ever greater degrees of complexity. Only the isolated signifier is not bound to other signifiers and therefore does not produce meaning.

It is important that the analysts do not skip over meaning. They should learn Freud and early Lacan; they should know how to interpret hidden meaning, signifiers linked in semantic chains and logical formulas. Yet there are texts in which words behave like names, like letters: units that do not rest upon other signifiers, but upon jouissance. This is the referent of the single word. Like the name of a beloved that provokes a response, like a curse, like a cry. In such cases the analyst does not interpret, he points to the hold that this sequence of sounds has on the body's enjoyment, and from there on the subject's effects and on the construction of his reality.

Sound. *Lalangue* in Lacan's conceptualization is the basic layer of the signifier: the sensory wave that carries it, the sound itself. If a poem calls for music more than a story does, it is for this reason. In infancy, sound was the only component of language. Language begins with a baby's babbling, which is only later charged with meaning, but before meaning, *lalangue* is the mouth's enjoyment of itself through the production of sounds. A simple example of listening to jouissance as it appears in sound would be a patient saying, "I hate that ssstinky guy," while drawing out the sibilant: ssss…tinky. Desire could be interpreted here as an allusion to the man's animality, especially if the smell of an animal had appeared elsewhere in the associations; but if one wants to draw attention to jouissance, one simply points to it. This can be done by stressing the signifier…ssss, or even by saying plainly: "There's enjoyment in your words." The effect of such a gesture can be that the patient begins to doubt the story that holds his anger in place and sees the anger itself as a mode of enjoyment. In that case, release from the symptom does not depend on grasping its meaning, but on recognizing jouissance and with that, the possibility of letting it go.

Just as Lévi-Strauss showed that language is not only spoken language, *lalangue* is not confined to speech either. As the gaze is not limited to the eye, it can appear in the ear, in eavesdropping, so too sound is the material of the phoneme, yet it may also be made of body parts and movement, tactile sensations, or other senses. These are the material elements that enter the mold of language. *Lalangue* is made of sensory fragments, not only of sound. The language of dance uses fragments of *lalangue* made of movement; the language of erotic life, of couplings and positions, uses an alphabet of partial gazes on a body.

Each of these layers, myth, narrative, turns of phrase, the formula of meaning, the isolated signifier, and sound, is an aspect of the patient's speech that calls for listening. A theory of the different aspects of meaning is like a set of hearing devices tuned to different frequencies of complexity. For the analyst, to be a poem is to dwell in language in all its Symbolic and Real dimensions.

Topology

To articulate the passage from meaning to the knotting of saying and jouissance, Lacan turns to topology: a branch of mathematics concerned with the properties of bodies. Do they have holes, cuts, edges, dimensions, networks, twists, knots? Can one give them a visual form? A mathematical formulation? Lacan made extensive use of topology, among other reasons, to formulate the paradoxical relations between the Symbolic order and the Real.

The topology that Lacan subverts is the topology that guided Freud in building psychoanalytic theory, the three-dimensional spheres. The Freudian ego has the shape of a three-dimensional bubble, like a cell membrane that defines the individual by its boundaries against the environment. Even the threat posed by knowledge of the repressed drive is experienced by the ego as an external threat. Freud's topographical model as well; conscious, pre-conscious, unconscious, rests on the topology of layered three-dimensional bodies, while the dynamic model describes the modes of movement between those layers.

The topology that guided Lévi-Strauss was that of networks. Structuralism began as a network mapping of motifs in myths. As the theory developed, he described the range of semantic linkages, from the quartet of meaning up to myth itself, as diagrams of nodes and connections. Network thinking was also a starting point for Lacan; yet unlike Freud and Lévi-Strauss, for Lacan topology was a deliberate way of thinking the psyche outside the fixations of three-dimensional space.

For Lacan, topology was a way of inventing theory. In his view, topological figures do not describe reality. Reality in any case does not exist with an independent ontological status but rather make possible forms of constructing reality. And it is precisely the taken-for-granted three-dimensionality of common sense that these forms are put into question.

Here is one example of Lacan's use of topology in the formulation of concepts. The notion of the uncanny, the intimate foreigner, a threat felt as coming from outside while it comes from within, can be described more adequately when the surface on which one marks the difference between inside and outside is a torus whose center lies outside it, rather than a sphere. The paradoxical relations between concepts such as conscious and unconscious, subject and Other, desire and jouissance, are expressed more fully when the opposition between them appears on the two "sides" of a Möbius strip, which also inscribes the continuity between them. The Borromean knot is a topological body that expresses reality as an interplay among three orders: as a three-legged stand stands only through the mutual support of its legs, so the Borromean knot produces reality through the knotting of the three registers together.

The late Lacanian approach brings the patient to a knot; an anchoring in the signifiers with which he identifies, which function for him as an anchor of being. In Lacan's terms, this is the sinthome: the particular weave in which the reality of the speaking being is bound.

Almost every theoretical development of Lacan was demonstrated in a topological figure; and what is most relevant to the passage from the Symbolic unconscious to the Real unconscious is the topology of the act: the subversive image of the cut that creates the surface on which it is made.

Act

An act is something the subject does in the course of which he disappears and emerges again. Insofar as the subject is held by identifications with signifiers, an act is an exit from a signifying system that sustains a subject, and a re-entry into a symbolic network on the other side of the act. It is a fateful choice: the subject is required to wager on who he will be on the far side. Resigning, enlisting, giving birth, or any deed that counts as an act to the extent that the subject becomes someone he does not yet know, someone who adopts or creates new coordinates by which he can exist as a figure in a story. The cut that fundamentally changes the surface on which it is made; that is the act the subject performs in a way that changes himself at the root.

Lacan's own passage from the Symbolic unconscious to the Real unconscious is an act: a destabilization of basic assumptions. Lacan wishes the analysand not to experience himself as a form. The cut casts doubt on the imaginary completeness of the ego as a three-dimensional sphere in Freud's topographical model. Structuralism, too, has an almost imaginary completeness in its aesthetic; yet Lacan does not only distance himself from the structuralism of his earlier position, but he also suspects the psychic motivations behind this kind of thinking, the use of the Symbolic and the Imaginary as a defense against the Real, a defense that can constrict being.

In his book, *The Marks of a Psychoanalysis* (Izcovich 2017), Louis Izcovich brings in the poet Borges to clarify what Lacan is trying to say about the dis-identification from signifying coordinates and being in the Real unconscious. In the parable in which Zhuangzi dreams he is a butterfly, the butterfly functions as a totem of identification, a signifier that forges links with other signifiers and thereby produces meaning. The effect of the signifier is so powerful that even if the represented and the representation were reversed, and it was the butterfly dreaming itself as Zhuangzi, there would still be no escape from the network of signifiers. The way Borges articulates the position beyond identifications is by imagining waking in the morning as a butterfly that knows nothing at all of Zhuangzi. This is a position from which the analyst operates when he lends him or herself as a medium for the act to take place.

Beyond the Pleasure Principle

The idea that the Symbolic can reduce being stands behind Lacan's reading of "Beyond the Pleasure Principle" (Freud 1920). The essay splits Freud's teaching into a "before" and an "after." Before, there is still an optimism that reading the signifiers of the unconscious will lead to cure. After, it becomes clear that interpretation is not enough. The death drive, in all its forms, persists. The myth that reconciles Freud to the fact that humanity's fate is to live with the death drive, is a metaphysical myth: the death drive as a biological, molecular, and physical phenomenon. The death drive is entropy; the tendency of matter to disintegrate, and in the Freudian myth, even the wish to disintegrate. If in the biblical version we are dust and to dust we return, in Freud it is dust's desire to return to itself. Freud builds a structure of different levels of complexity whose collapse is the work of the death drive, while the energy required to pay for building higher complexities is the life drive, experienced, indeed, as effort, in contrast to the lazy nirvana of the death drive.

Lacan subverts Freud's metaphysics and the anchoring of the human in the cosmic. This is the imaginary, animistic stance to which Lacan objects. For Lacan there is a sharp cut between the human and everything else, because the human speaks. Only human beings have language, and language is the source of the death drive. As speaking beings, humans have a singular fate by which the death drive must be understood. The death drive is the effect of the signifier. Lacan treats Freud's motivation to hold on to metaphysical beliefs with a certain indulgence; it is the human weakness for structure, the mark of the signifier afflicting Freud too.

The death drive first appears as a signifier that disrupts harmony, at least in the consciousness of the subject, who is already the product of the signifier. The word "kills" the thing when it replaces it; and for that reason, at first the death drive is identified with the signifier. The word stands in the place of the thing. The word establishes the principle of exchange that allows other words to replace one another. This principle of exchange is paid for by the loss of the Real thing. One striking figure of such a refusal can be found in elective mutism. They resist the effect of the signifier, the invitation to identify with the symbolic world.

From the moment the human being identifies with the signifier, and identifies as the subject whose existence is assumed in light of the desire produced by signifiers, the death drive changes sides. The subject's desire hides from itself the fact that it is a product of language, of the Other. Whoever was there before the signifier, before intention was retroactively attributed, gets sealed outside the creation of language, as if the linguistic creature, closed in a phantasmatic, topological way, had been there from the beginning.

The subject as a creature of language experiences drives as a death drive: as the threat that the links between signifiers will break, the links that hold the subject as meaning. Should one identify or not identify, or to what extent identify, with the subject who lives in language, defined by the Other; or with the speaking being, enjoying, particular, not completely in language? This is an ethical question: what is psychoanalysis' position with respect to Symbolic and Real identifications?

Ethics

In "Civilization and Its Discontents," Freud says that the aim of psychoanalysis is to reduce the damages of civilization (Freud 1930). What Freud had in mind was the weakening of the superego's shame and guilt. Lacan takes up this ethical orientation and asks: what civilization is it whose damages we must overcome? Is it western culture, as Margaret Mead criticized it for suffocating the puritan subject and making him neurotic, while romanticizing the "natives"? For Lévi-Strauss, civilization is precisely the remedy. Structure sustains the subject, and the threat is that the myth, and with it the subject, might collapse.

As we saw in topology, so too in ethics, Lacan, in a subversive move, cuts the surface on which he is working, overturning the very theory from which his thought emerged. Within structuralism, the subject exists as a hypothesis: an assumed, hypothetical subject, the structuralist subject who is passive with respect to the chain of signifiers that determines him without his awareness. What does not appear in structuralism is the drive, the human being as an enjoying entity, present not as spoken-about but as speaking. Here is an example that illustrates this, mentioned in Chapter 2. A child says something witty. Everyone laughs. The child enjoys their laughter; he reads it as an attribution of an intention to make them laugh. The attribution of intention produces the function of intention. An intention to amuse awakens in him as if it was re-awakened, and he repeats the gesture once more.

Is that all we should expect ourselves to be, entities whose existence is merely assumed? Lacan wanted, for the analysand, a more Real existence than that of the subject. He called it the speaking being. This is a movement from the question "What do I want?" to the utterance "That's me!" The structural, mythic, metaphysical conception, the complexity of meaning itself, can be experienced as what prevents anything other than the subject from existing at all.

A Clinic of Subversion

Subversion is a complex kind of overturning. There are two movements here: in Latin *sub*, a position "under," and *vertere*, "to turn." Like a wrestler who slips under his opponent in order to flip him; like a nucleus within a social movement that gnaws at its foundations and takes it over. In logic, the expression of subversion would be a destabilization of basic assumptions. For Lacan it was a passion. In his professional psychoanalytic affiliations, Lacan again and again unsettled the establishment's mechanisms of certification and normalization.

In Lacan's teaching the subversions follow each other in succession. One example is that Lacan illustrates the exit from imaginary identification through subversion with the diagram of the mirror stage (Lacan ([1953–1954] 1991). The axis on which the mirror turns reveals it as a mirror and wakes the subject from the illusion that his image is himself. Another example is that Lacan points out that the Cartesian subject of self-consciousness had to exist so that Freud could subvert it and invent the unconscious. Lacan also unsettles the subject of the unconscious itself, a mythical creature whose existence is assumed as an agent of desire. Instead, Lacan points at the dimension of saying that subverts what is said.

The crucial subversion in Lacan's late clinic is between the Symbolic and the Real, between knowledge and jouissance. This is not a movement of "understanding more," that is, an elaboration of the myth one lives in, but a movement of changing place. Instead of demanding a guarantee of existence through meaning in the Other, one identifies with the jouissance at the heart of the symptom. The role of interpretation is to undermine knowledge, not explanations that close it. When the patient arrives with a sentence he already "knows why," that is precisely the problem. Will he dare to know less and to be more, to enjoy?

Subversion occurs in the clinic when analysis succeeds in illuminating the jouissance at the heart of the disturbance and in stirring an identification with it. Late Lacan undergoes a further shift in identification: from the Imaginary of ego psychology, through the Symbolic of early Lacan, to a new definition of who "I" am. The Real I, is the one who exists through the act of speech. As was said in the section on the topology of the act, the act is a cut that creates the surface on which it is made. The subject who has given up the fantasy of existing in the gaze of the Other speaks himself into existence. The analyst's task is to notice the emergence of this identity and to link the patient to it by saying, "That's you!"; to transfer the authority over reality back to him by saying "That's how you say it!," and inviting him, to own the core of his being by saying: "this is your singular enjoyment."

Here is a clinical example. A patient reported that many of the goals of treatment have been achieved, yet her excess weight and her difficulty keeping a diet have not moved at all. She wonders whether she should accept herself as she is. The identification we spoke about shifts: from identification with body image and the thought that she should accept how she looks, to identification with the drive, to identify with the one who so enjoyed eating. She identified as an enjoying being. The result of making this identification possible was less necessity to eat, and weight loss. As long as the enjoying identity was repudiated, jouissance spoke through the act of eating. Respect for the drive, and identification as an enjoying entity, are part of the solution; but no less important is the entity that declares itself into existence and says, "This is me!"

The speaking being speaks its enjoying being into existence. That is what it does when it says, "This is me," and Lacan emphasizes the act of saying, the position from which she determines who she is. There lies the being of enunciation.

To illustrate the difference between the subject of the statement and the being of enunciation, Lacan brings in the liar paradox. When a person says, "I am lying," is he lying or telling the truth? If he is telling the truth, then it is true that he is lying; and if he is not telling the truth about lying, then he is telling the truth. Had he said, "You are lying," there would be no paradox, since it is entirely possible that he is telling the truth when he says of someone else that he is lying. What is the mistaken, narrow assumption that produces the paradox? And what do we need to bring into our field of vision for the paradox to disappear? The mistaken assumption is that the liar is one person, whereas in the utterance "You are lying" there are two, one who speaks and one who appears in the statement. The solution to the paradox, then, lies in distinguishing between the speaker, who says, "I am lying," and the signifier "I," which appears in the sentence "I am lying." At the beginning of treatment, the patient identifies with the subject of the statement. This is a process of liberation from identification with imaginary images and symbolic roles, and identification with the Real kernel of the symptom.

Late Lacan would ask about the possibility of sustaining being on the basis of a jouissance tied to the solitary signifier. Not the fantasy of a big Other embodied in a parental figure, who guarantees meanings and will save him, but the opposite; the certainty that the Other does not exist, and that one ought to stop waiting for him to arrive. At the beginning of analysis, the analyst occupies the place of the one to whom knowledge is attributed, which allows one to believe that there is something to know, as if the analysand's aim were to be known, to be the one thought about, to be registered in the gaze of the Other, so that self-knowledge would be guaranteed by a supposed knower, as with Descartes.

In early Lacan, existence as a desiring subject is a worthy aim. In late Lacan, satisfaction takes precedence. The shedding of the subject in favor of the speaking being is a rescue from an endless metonymic desire, where words replace one another forever without reaching the thing. The solitary signifier makes satisfaction possible. Enjoyment in the Real. There is a preference of the Real over truth, and of being over logic.

To conclude

The book has followed one question, returning in each chapter in a different guise: how human beings exist in language. How they gain existence through myths, through institutions, through narratives, through symptoms that hold meaning for them even when they suffer. The clinic of the Symbolic, in Freud's reading, under Lévi-Strauss's inspiration, and in early Lacan, is not "interpretation" alone but an ethics: one that allows the subject to be woven into culture, to be at home in the structures that sustain him, to hold a singular destiny within a shared network.

The limit of meaning can become clearer: there are instances when interpretation adds knowledge and changes nothing; there are times when explanation itself becomes a defense; and there is an insistence of jouissance and repetition, what Freud encountered as the move beyond the pleasure principle, that does not submit to clarification. From here, late Lacan's turn is not an "abandonment" of the Symbolic but its subversion: a listening that does not settle for meaning but hears a tying, attention to the solitary letter, to *lalangue*, to the materiality of speech, to the way a body enjoys a signifier and, in that enjoyment, conceals itself.

So, there is no choice here between a "right" clinic and a "wrong" one, but a movement: from myth to poem, from the network to the hole, from knowledge to the point of jouissance that holds the symptom. And precisely here the concluding principle arrives; one needs to be a subject to undergo a subversion into a speaking being, just as affirmation takes place before negation. This is the process of analysis: to allow the emergence of the desiring subject, only for it to become clear how much he is assumed by the Other, which opens the possibility for a subversion of the identification of the subject, not only as a figure in a myth, but as an enjoying being who speaks himself into existence.

References

Freud, S. (1920). Beyond the pleasure principle. In J. Strachey (Ed. & Trans.), *The standard edition of the complete psychological works of Sigmund Freud* (Vol. 18, pp. 7–64). Hogarth Press.

Freud, S. (1930). Civilization and its discontents. In J. Strachey (Ed. & Trans.), *The standard edition of the complete psychological works of Sigmund Freud* (Vol. 21, pp. 59–145). Hogarth Press.

Izcovich, L. (2017). *The marks of a psychoanalysis.* Karnac.

Lacan, J. ([1953–1954] 1991). *The seminar of Jacques Lacan. Book I: Freud's papers on technique, 1953–1954* (J.-A. Miller, Ed., J. Forrester, Trans.). W. W. Norton & Company.

Lacan, J. ([1964–1965] 1977). *The seminars of Jacques Lacan. Book 11: The four fundamental concepts of psychoanalysis.* Norton.

List of Myths

Index

Note: Locators in *italic* and **bold** refer figures and tables respectively, and locators followed by "n" refer end notes.

For Product Safety Concerns and Information please contact our EU representative GPSR@taylorandfrancis.com
Taylor & Francis Verlag GmbH, Kaufingerstraße 24, 80331 München, Germany

www.ingramcontent.com/pod-product-compliance
Ingram Content Group UK Ltd.
Pitfield, Milton Keynes, MK11 3LW, UK
UKHW022019180926
475701UK00005B/925

9781041302889